Dr Geoffrey Leader & Lucille Leader

PARKINSON'S DISEASE

Reducing Symptoms

with **nutrition**

and **drugs**

Third Edition

Foreword by Professor Leslie Findley
Consultant Neurologist Medical Advisor to
The European Parkinson's Disease Association

British Library Cataloguing in Publication Data. A catalogue record for this book is
available from the British Library.

American Library of Congress Cataloguing in Publication Data

Published by Denor Press Limited
Email: denorgroup@gmail.com
Website: www.denorpress.com

Book Cover Design by Jonathan Phillips
www.toccatadesign.com

Layout & Publishers Services
Commercial Campaigns www.commercialcampaigns.co.uk

Printed by Lightning Source/Ingram
www.lightningsource.co.uk

To the Memory of Dr Erich Segal, Tom Isaacs, Dr Joseph Orden and Philip Leader for scientific inspiration

To People with Parkinson's Disease and their devoted Caregivers

Special Acknowledgements

Dr Erich Segal and Karen Segal, for continuing inspiration.

Professor Leslie Findley, Consultant Neurologist, for his excellent Foreword to this book, for his erudition and unstinting support.

Dr David Perlmutter and Helen Kimber, for their important contributions to this volume.

Tom Isaacs for his generous contribution to this book and the inspiration that he is to all.

Dr Lynn Toohey, Dr T. Michael Culp, Sue Jones, Nicole Golembo, Kate Neil and Christopher Astill-Smith for helpful research information.

Dr Serena Leader, for editing and encouragement.

Sevim Osman, for copy editing at Denor Press and immense patience.

Alison Kiersz-Brownstone, Natasha Crombie, Enio Qirko and Nicholas Stapleton at Denor Press, for indexing and editorial services.

Beverley Friedgood and Veronica Nixon, for editorial services.

Jean Harding, for moral support.

Mary Baker OBE, Founder of the European Parkinson's Disease Association and Jo Rosen, Founder of the Parkinson's Resource Orgnaisation USA, for encouragement.

Lizzie Graham, for continued support from The European Parkinson's Disease Association.

David Uri, psychotherapist and hypnotherapist, for patient psychology.

Rae Leader for culinary expertise.

Esther Orden, for 'sound boarding', support and encouragement.

Joe Leader and Jacqui Taylor for great support.

Felicia Beder, for promotional services.

Brendan Beder, Stella Beder and Edna Freinkel for promotion.

Morris Orden and Elizabeth Davis for assistance and moral support.

Richard Conway, for promotion.

The Highgate Hospital Staff, for caring co-operation.

DISCLAIMER AND CAUTIONARY NOTE

The recommendations in this book are not intended to replace general medical advice or the advice of a neurologist, nutritionist, dietician, clinical biochemist, pathologist, pharmacist, psychologist, surgeon, anaesthesiologist, dentist, occupational therapist, nurse, physiotherapist, exercise therapist or any other healthcare professional.

Medical knowledge is constantly expanding. As new clinical experience and experimental knowledge is gained, management needs to be constantly re-evaluated and updated.

Patient individuality makes it imperative for supervision by healthcare professionals at all times. As such, the publisher, editors and authors cannot accept liability for any problems arising directly or indirectly from the application of the advice contained herein.

Contents

About the Authors

Lucille Leader Dip ION MBANT NTCC CNHC Reg

Email: denorgroup@gmail.com

Lucille Leader, Nutritional Therapist, practices at The Highgate Hospital in London. Her experience includes being the Nutrition Director of the London Pain Relief and Nutritional Support Clinic at The Highgate Hospital. This clinic was an early pioneer in the integrated, team approach to the management of chronic illness, with a special interest in the management of Parkinson's Disease and Multiple Sclerosis.
She is particularly interested in the biochemically-based nutritional support of patients with neurological degenerative disease, particularly Parkinson's Disease.

She is author, co-author and editor of other successful books including: **Parkinson's Disease Dopamine Metabolism, Applied Biochemistry and Nutrition** ISBN-13: 978-0-9526056-6-9 (Denor Press)
Parkinson's Disease Top Tips to Optimize Function ISBN-13: 978-0956172235 (Denor Press)
Parkinson's Disease – The Way Forward! ISBN: 0 9526056 8 6 (Denor Press)
Morbo Di Parkinson – Suggerimenti Nutrizionali (Pythagora Press, Milan, Italy) with Professors Aroldo Rossi and Lia Rossi Prosperi ISBN: 88 85852 31 9
Medical Collaboration for Nutritional Therapists: (Denor Press) ISBN: 978 0 9526056 5 2
Lectureships have included the Nutritional Therapy MSc degree course at CNELM (accredited Middlesex University, UK), BSc courses at Westminster University and the Institute of Optimum Nutrition, in the UK

She has delivered many lectures on the nutritional aspects in Parkinson's Disease to Parkinson's Disease support groups in The United Kingdom, South Africa, Austria, Croatia and the United States of America. She has also lectured to health professionals and has been interviewed by the BBC and SABC Radios. She has published in medical, para-medical, nutritional and health support journals including the European Parkinson's Disease Association (EPDA), The Motor Disorders Journal, The EPNN (Nurses) Journal and that of The Parkinson's Society of the Czech Republic

Parkinson's Disease Congress presentations include:
The World Parkinson's Congress in Scotland, Meeting of the Minds Congress in the USA, The Parkinson's Disease Congress for Nutrition and Sexuality in Vienna, The European Parkinson's Disease (EPDA) Congresses in Italy, Portugal and Croatia and in London.
Lucille Leader was honoured with a Quality of Life Award for Parkinson's in The United States and the CAM Outstanding Practice Award for the UK.

Lucille Leader is a Fellow of The Royal Society of Medicine in London, UK and a member of it's Food and Health Council. Memberships include the British Association for Applied Nutrition and Nutritional Therapy (BANT), CNHC, and The British Society for Ecological Medicine. She is also a member of the The European Parkinson's Disease (EPDA) Expert Review Panel.

Dr Geoffrey Leader MB ChB FRCA

Email: denorgroup@gmail.com

Dr Geoffrey Leader, a graduate of the Royal College of Anaesthetists in London, is a Consultant Anaesthesiologist and posts include that of Medical Director of The London Pain Relief and Nutritional Support Clinic at The Highgate Hospital in London. He is a leading pioneer in the multi-disciplinary management of chronic illness and pain mnanagement. The special interest of his Clinic has been the optimization of functional health in people with Parkinson's Disease.

Dr Geoffrey Leader has held senior academic posts internationally. In the UK he was Chairman of the Anaesthetic Department, Head of Intensive Care and Pain Clinic at Newham General Hospital, London and Senior Lecturer and Honorary Senior Consultant at The Royal London Hospital Medical College. In South Africa he held academic appointments at Natal and Witwatersrand Universities and in The Netherlands at The University of Erasmus. He is co-author and editor of other successful books:
Parkinson's Disease Dopamine Metabolism, Applied Biochemistry and Nutrition ISBN-13: 978-0-9526056-6-9 (Denor Press)
Parkinson's Disease Top Tips to Optimize Function ISBN-13: 978-0956172235 (Denor Press)
Parkinson's Disease – The Way Forward! ISBN: 0 9526056 8 6 (Denor Press)
Morbo Di Parkinson – Suggerimenti Nutrizionali (Pythagora Press, Milan, Italy) with Professors Aroldo Rossi and Lia Rossi Prosperi ISBN: 88 85852 31 9

Dr Geoffrey Leader is particularly interested in the intravenous nutritional support of patients with Parkinson's Disease as well as the specialised details of their management during anaesthesia and sedation including detoxification from anaesthetic drugs. He has presented papers on anaesthetic subjects at international congresses and has published in prestigious anaesthetic journals including Anaesthesia and Dutch anaesthetic journals. His Parkinson's Disease Congress presentations include:

"The Intravenous Aspects of Nutritional Support in Parkinson's Disease" at the Parkinson's Disease Congress for Nutrition and Sexuality in Vienna.
"Nutritional Therapy and Cellular Environment in Parkinson's Disease" at the ground-breaking Parkinson's symposium "Meeting of the Minds" in the United States.
"Specialised Nutritional Management in Parkinson's Disease" at the 5th Multi-disciplinary Conference of the European Parkinson's Disease Association (EPDA) in Portugal.

He was honoured in the United States with a "Quality of Life Award for Parkinson's". Dr Geoffrey Leader is a Fellow of both the Royal College of Anaesthetists and The Royal Society of Medicine in the United Kingdom and a Member of the British Society of Ecological Medicine.

Professor Leslie Findley KLJ TD MD FRCP FACP

E-mail: ljfindley@uk-consultants.co.uk

Professor Leslie Findley is Professor of Health Sciences (Neurology) at South Bank University, London, UK. He also holds the position of Senior Consultant Neurologist at the Essex Neurosciences Unit, Oldchurch Hospital, Romford, Essex, UK.

Professor Findley is Founder and Chairman of the National Tremor Foundation and a Trustee of the National ME Centre for Fatigue Syndromes. He is a member of the Medical Advisory Panel of the European Parkinson's Disease Association (EPDA.) As past Chairman of The Parkinson's Disease Society of the United Kingdom, he is currently its Honorary Vice President. He is a member of the WHO Working Party on Parkinson's Disease.

Professor Findley is a promoter of the multi-disciplinary approach to the management of Parkinson's Disease. He has written the Foreword to the well- acclaimed book on the subject of this integrated approach, "Parkinson's Disease – The Way Forward!" together with Dr Geoffrey Leader, Lucille Leader, Professor Aroldo Rossi, Dr Lia Rossi-Prosperi and other eminent specialists in the field of Parkinson's Disease. His main clinical and research interests are movement disorders and fatigue syndromes.

Contributors

Tom Isaacs BSc (Hons) MRICS

E-mail: www.cureparkinsons.org.uk

Tom Isaacs contributed the chapter "I used to be a nutritional 'neurosceptic'......."
A successful chartered surveyor, he developed Parkinson's Disease at an early age.
He has raised considerable funds for Parkinson's Disease research. Tom Isaacs was UK's "Charity Personality of the Year" and co-founded The Cure Parkinson's Trust, UK.

David Perlmutter MD FACN ABIHM

Dr. Perlmutter is a Board-Certified Neurologist, Fellow of the American College of Nutrition and four-time *New York Times* bestselling author including the #1 NYT bestseller *Grain Brain. H*e has published extensively in peer-reviewed scientific journals including *Archives of Neurology* and *The Journal of Applied Nutrition. Lecture presentations include* Columbia and Harvard Universities amongst other medical institutions. His many awards include *The Linus Pauling Award, Clinician of the Year*Award and *Humanitarian of the Year* Award. He is Associate Professor at the University of Miami Miller School of Medicine.

Helen Kimber BSc (Hons) MSc PGCE ECNP

 A graduate of Nutrition from Huddersfield and Surrey Universities and well- known academic lecturer, Helen Kimber has contributed to the section on Liver Detoxification Guidelines. She has contributed to the formulation of various nutritional supplements.

Foreword

Professor Leslie J Findley KLJ TD MD F RCP FACP

Professor of Health Sciences (Neurology), Southbank Univerity, London UK.
Consultant Neurologist, Essex Neurosciences Unit, Romford, Essex UK

Parkinson's disease affects at least 6 million people worldwide. Although recognised as a condition affecting the older age ranges, 1:10 patients are diagnosed before the age of 50. With an aging population, the number of people with neurodegenerative disorders, such as Parkinson's disease, is expected to rise steadily. It represents a major contributor to chronic morbidity in every community.

Despite the fact that Parkinson's disease is a progressive neurological disorder of unknown cause and, as yet, has no known cure, modern medical management, especially with dopaminergic medications in their various forms, does allow, for many, good control of the motor symptoms of the disorder. *This is being refined by the simultaneous application of biochemically based nutritional management aimed at optimising the positive effects of drugs and minimising distressing side-effects. As such, with good medical management, the individual with Parkinson's disease may have a normal, or near normal, life expectancy.*

In the last two decades there has been a growing awareness of the non-motor symptoms which may significantly impair the quality of life of those with Parkinson's disease. Such symptoms may include, amongst others, psychological symptoms, bowel dysfunction and lack of energy. Indeed, it has also now become recognised, as with other neurodegenerative disorders, that the major contributor to lack of quality of life in Parkinson's disease, is the mood, emotional status and personal attitude of the individual.

This increased awareness of the complexity of Parkinson's disease has been associated with an increase in the variability and complexity of treatments offered. It is widely accepted that the simple "doctor-drug" model of treatment is no longer sufficient to give that quality of care that one may expect in the modern era.

The complexity of treatments required can best be delivered in the form of a multi-disciplinary team approach to provide holistic and comprehensive management for Parkinson's disease. This ensures the input of skills necessary to the individual to maintain optimum health, both physical and mental, and thereby a good quality of life. *An important member of the multi-disciplinary team is the nutritionist as optimum nutrition, both general and therapeutic, is a "keystone" to any long-term management strategy.*

This timely volume is directed to those with Parkinson's disease, their carers and health professionals. It provides an accessible and scientifically referenced source of information on the diverse aspects of drugs and nutrition. It covers theoretical concepts of good nutritional management, the effects of nutrition on general health and energy. Additionally, it presents the interplay and possible interactions between diet and drugs, and inevitably extends into the more general advice on "good health practice" for those with parkinsonism.

The authors are experienced, and renowned, practising clinical nutritionists. They are advocates for the nutritional approach to improving functional health in neuro-degenerative disorders in general, *and Parkinson's disease specifically.*

Hippocrates, more than 2,000 years ago stated:

"Make food your medicine".

It is fair to say that he did not have access to modern medications. I would humbly suggest if he was to write that aphorism today, he would probably say:

"Make food *part* of your medicine".

In this volume, Lucille and Geoffrey Leader have done just that.

Professor Leslie Findley

"I used to be a nutritional 'neurosceptic'..."

by Tom Isaacs

So what is this strange word "nutrition?" On its own it is a lifeless, rather dull word - a bit like "nice," only for food. It conjures up thoughts of cereal packets and health food stores, of self-imposed dietary regimes and taking things "in moderation." In short, it does not convey the most profound of messages.

It certainly does not even hint at its true definition or its true worth in the overall scheme of things. But delve beneath the surface of the word "nutrition," and you suddenly realize you are dealing with the materials for the maintenance of all life. Without adequate nutrition, we die. With nutrition, we shape our own physical and mental characteristics in a constant cycle of decay and renewal. This process is embodied in the maxim "we are what we eat."

But what has nutrition got to do with Parkinson's Disease?

I was the biggest "nutritional neurosceptic" of all. Certainly, if "I was what I ate," I would look like a cross between a potato and a family- sized bar of milk chocolate! Surely the only thing I could then do to treat my Parkinson's would be to "keep taking the pills!"

How hopelessly naive? How wrong can you be?

It is nearly 10 years ago since I was diagnosed with "Parkinson's". The first year after diagnosis was the worst. It took me that long to get my head round it. I came to understand that I would have to live my life by a new set of rules. There were times when I had a very real sense of how Parkinson's had the potential to take away my freedom. I therefore became determined to live my life out of sight of the perimeter fences. And that is what this book is about. It's about maintaining the boundaries of Parkinson's at an acceptable distance.

It achieves this by analyzing the biochemistry of each individual and addressing nutritional deficiency or excess using diet and/or supplements. It considers the interaction between drugs and food. But that is not all. The book also covers important and often overlooked topics such as bowel function and the management of adrenalin and stress which affect the production of our own dopamine resources. The result of all these things is improved well-being and a reduction of distressing symptoms.

To me, nutrition is now the most important method of managing my health. It is a discipline which forms the platform for all other contributory factors to my well-being; factors such as drug therapy, physiotherapy, exercise and of course, common sense.

It all seems so obvious to me now. Whereas my neurologist succeeds in adapting my brain function *after* its invasion and subsequent occupation by Parkinson's, nutrition is like my *own* resistance force. It makes my body as inhospitable as possible for Parkinson's to coexist with the rightful inhabitants of my brain. When the cure comes, I will be ready. Vive la resistance!

Lucille and Geoffrey Leader are at the cutting edge of Parkinson's nutritional, clinical evaluation. They have also been in the front line of my own battle with the condition. With their help I have been able to live a life, since diagnosis, which has been as rewarding as it has been punishing; as fulfilling as much as it has seemed unfair. I have been incredibly fortunate to have them as counsellors and as friends. With just a small investment of time and discipline, you will reap the benefits of their indefatigable enthusiasm and knowledge of a poorly understood subject.

The protocols in this book are not based on hearsay, rumor or unsubstantiated theory. They are based on hard scientific evidence and fact. To anyone touched by Parkinson's, I commend this book to you. To anyone with Parkinson's itself, this is an indispensable tool to help you to help yourself. Don't be a "nutritional neurosceptic" like I was. Read on and reap the benefits!

Tom Isaacs BSc (Hons) MRICS

Tom Isaacs, a successful chartered surveyer, was diagnosed with Parkinson's disease at the young age of 27. Since 1999 he has raised over £400,000 for Parkinson's Disease research projects. Having already raised £40,000 completing a 1250 mile walk from John O'Groats to Lands End, he left his job as a Director of a London property company in 2002 to undertake his "Coastin'" challenge. Between April 2002 and April 2003, Tom walked 4,500 miles around the coastline of Britain, climbed the highest mountains in England, Scotland and Wales and ran the Flora London Marathon, with the aim of raising funds and to help build awareness and understanding of the disease. During that year, Tom met representatives from over 90 Parkinson's Disease groups around the coast, gave more than 190 interviews to local and national media and walked with more than 40 MPs, 9 Mayors, and 16 celebrities. Tom was runner-up in the GMTV/Daily Mirror Fundraiser of the Year Award 2004. He is currently UK's "Charity Personality of the Year" and is the co-founder of The Cure Parkinson's Trust, UK. Website: www.cureparkinsons.org.uk

Chapter 1

How Specialised Nutrition Influences Drug Response & Functional Health

Nutrition and General Cellular Function

The influence of nutrition on functional health in Parkinson's Disease is widespread. Bearing in mind that all cellular function is dependent on the adequate nutritional status of cells, this influence must surely be vital in the management of chronic illness.

Vitamin C deficiency may cause scurvy. Deficiency of vitamin B1 can be linked with beriberi, iron with anaemia, essential fatty acids with inflammatory disease and calcium with osteoporosis. Similarly, dopamine deficiency may lead to Parkinson's Disease.

Dopamine is metabolized from dietary protein. Therefore, deficiencies of digestive and other enzymes and their co-enzymes (dietary vitamins and minerals including zinc, folate, iron, vitamin B6) necessary for dopamine metabolism, may compromise this metabolic pathway and further amplify the degenerative process.

Cellular energy can be compromised in Parkinson's Disease. Research has demonstrated that, whilst essential, L-dopa administration may also compromise energy metabolism. It would therefore be pertinent to support the energy cycle (citric acid cycle).

This cycle is dependent on glucose (from fruit, vegetables and grains or medium chain triglycerides from coconut oil together with specific nutrients (including vitamin B1, vitamin B2, vitamin B3, vitamin B5, vitamin C, NADH, co-enzyme Q10, biotin, magnesium malate, iron and copper), obtained from dietary sources and therapeutic nutritional supplementation.

Mood, energy and restful sleep are often dependent on a balanced blood sugar resulting from a better-timed and appropriate diet.

Inflammatory and anti-inflammatory cellular responses are controlled by hormones which are dependent on zinc, vitamin B6 and other nutrients as co-enzymes.

Nutrition and Absorption of Nutrients and Drugs

Bowel function is improved by sufficient fibre-containing foods (appropriate to neurological illness) and water. By optimising bowel function, the absorption of drugs and nutrients is facilitated.

Nutrition and Drug Efficacy

Specific metabolites of dietary protein, the 'neutral' amino acids, compete with the drug L-dopa for absorption from the intestine and again through the blood brain barrier. By manipulating the diet so as to avoid competition between these specific constituents of food and L-dopa, patients in our clinic notice that their drugs "kick-in" more efficiently. With drug-nutrient awareness, it is easier to monitor drug response and optimal timing of drug dosage and administration can be achieved. As such patients report that they experience less dyskinesia.

The drug monitoring schemes used in our clinic (L-dopa alone or in combination with other dopaminergic drugs) are presented in this book. They incorporate a diet compatible with optimal absorption of L-dopa as well as the appropriate timing of drug intake. Health professionals, patients and care givers are thereby helped to predict onset and duration of dopaminergic drugs. The application of this information has the potential to smooth out the "on-off" period.

By addressing nutritional deficiencies, supporting cellular energy and anti-inflammatory hormonal support, optimising bowel function and arranging the diet to be compatible with the absorption of L-dopa, some distressing symptoms experienced by people with Parkinson's Disease may be reduced.

Dr Geoffrey Leader & Lucille Leader

Chapter 2

Nutritional Therapy within the Multidisciplinary Team

It is now acknowledged that there is no "mono" therapy in the management of the diverse health problems associated with Parkinson's disease. Indeed, in 2005, the dynamic European Parkinson's Disease Association (EPDA) saw fit to convene a triumphant international congress in Lisbon, Portugal, to finally establish the much needed "integrated" approach to the management of this illness.

In a degenerative disease of this nature, various primary aspects of functional health need to be supported. As such, a core team of health professionals should ideally include the following:

Neurologist, General Practitioner, Nutritional Therapist, Speech Therapist, Physiotherapist, Osteopath, Remedial Movement Therapist, Remedial Masseur/se, Specialist Nurse, Sexual Therapist, Psychologist/Hypnotherapist, Autogenic Training Therapist. Other specialists may be consulted as needed for example, Gastroenterologist and Ear, Nose and Throat Specialist.

The potential of Nutritional Therapy in adjuvant medical care has been neglected in the past.

However, great strides have been made in biochemical analysis, resulting in increased levels of academic awareness. University degree courses in clinical nutrition have been established and consequently Nutritional Therapy is now recognised as an integral part of functional health care.

The influence of the Nutritional Therapist is comprehensive, underpinning the potential for other specialties. For example:

a) Drug-nutrient interactions must be addressed. In the authors' clinical experience, L-dopa medication is better absorbed and more efficacious if taken within a special dietary protocol, reducing side effects and dyskinesia. This enables other specialists to work more effectively with patients as they will be more likely to achieve improved levels of mobility.

b) Bowel function, frequently a problem in Parkinson's Disease, can be regulated by specialized dietary protocols.

c) Energy and blood sugar levels can be supported by nutritional manipulation.

d) Swallowing and chewing problems can be addressed by using specialized "predigested" foods, with or without tube feeding.

e) Intravenous nutritional support can be administered for mal- absorption.

f) Nutritional awareness can reduce exposure to harmful free radicals and environmental toxins. Antioxidant therapy is nutritionally based.

g) Nutritional biochemical assessments give an indication of cellular status and deficiencies. Given this detailed information, the degenerative process can be "supported" appropriately and the established cellular environment can be up or down-regulated. Digestive capability, intestinal permeability, allergy and food intolerances can be assessed and helpful recommendations made.

h) Some medications affect the nutritional status of cells. These effects can be monitored and appropriate supplementation provided.

i) "Peri-Surgical Nutrition" is now an established subject which enhances recovery from surgery and anaesthesia.

4

Chapter 3

Body Composition

What are human beings made of?

Our bodies contain many nutritional factors- **proteins, carbohydrates, fats, vitamins, minerals and water!** Too little or too much of these components may lead to ill health. Medical laboratories can measure an individual's nutritional status, both inside and outside the cells. Nutrients can be measured, for example, in blood, hair, sweat and urine. It is now possible to correct many of the imbalances found by dietary regulation and the administration of nutritional supplements.

What do proteins do?

Proteins are the "building blocks" of the body and perform many important functions:

Enzymes (catalysts which make things happen) are proteins and neurotransmitters (chemical messengers in the brain) are metabolized (formed) from protein. Dopamine is a neurotransmitter which is found to be deficient in Parkinson's Disease patients. It too is metabolized from dietary protein.

• Complete protein is contained in eggs, dairy produce, fish, poultry, meat and soy. Partial protein (not containing all the essential amino acids) is contained in pulses, grains and other food that can be combined to form complete protein.

Although soy is a complete protein, it is a lectin and not always suitable in neurological conditions.

What do carbohydrates do?

Each cell in the body needs and makes energy in order to perform its function. The body turns carbohydrates into glucose which is the main source of cellular energy production. Together with specific vitamins and minerals, this enables cells to generate energy during a process known as the Citric Acid Cycle (Krebs Cycle).

• Carbohydrates are contained in grains including wheat, buckwheat, rice, corn, millet and also in fruit and vegetables.

Note: Glucose utilisation can be a problem in Parkinson's disease. An alternative fuel source is found in coconut oil (medium chain triglycerides (MCTs)).

What do fats do?

There are many kinds of fats with different functions – including Saturated and Unsaturated Fats, Medium Chain Triglycerides (MCTs), Essential Fatty Acids (EFAs) and Mono- unsaturated Fats. Saturated Fat is a source of energy and forms a protective covering around organs and limbs. Cholesterol is essential to the formation of male and female hormones.. MCTs can be used as a cellular fuel source.

Cholesterol and EFAs are integral to all cell membranes including those of the brain (neurones) and also produce prostaglandins (hormones) which contribute to the control of inflammation

- Saturated fats are found in animal produce (meats, eggs, dairy), monounsaturated fat in olive or avocado oil and MCTs in coconut oil
- EFAs containing EPA (eicosapentanoic acid) are found in oily fish including sardines, herring, mackerel and salmon.
- EFAs containing GLA (gamma linoleic acid – Omega 6) are found in nuts and seeds including primrose and borage oils, almonds, sunflower and sesame seeds.

What do vitamins do?

Vitamins are organic substances necessary in the diet, in small quantities, for a variety of biochemical processes. Deficiencies can lead to disease such as beriberi (vit.B1) and scurvy (vit.C). Vitamins are either water or fat soluble (they dissolve in either fat or water in the diet, for their absorption). Functions include:

- Vitamin B6 needed in dopamine metabolism.
- Vitamin C needed for collagen formation and also the metabolism (formation) of noradrenaline (norepinephrine) from dopamine.
- Vitamins A, C and E needed as vital antioxidants.
- Some vitamins work in association with enzymes. They act as "co-enzymes" to facilitate enzyme activity.
- Significant amounts of vitamins are contained in fruit, vegetables and grains.

What do minerals do?

Minerals, inorganic substances obtained from the diet, are necessary for many cellular processes in the body. Deficiencies can lead to disease states such as osteoporosis (calcium) and anaemia (iron), as can excesses. "*Although people with Parkinson's Disease can demonstrate cellular deficiencies of specific minerals, there are regretfully contraindications to their administration as they have been shown in research to contribute to metabolic difficulties.*" Some examples of mineral functions include:

- Calcium, magnesium and phosphorous needed for bone formation.

- Calcium and magnesium also needed for muscle contraction and relaxation.

- Zinc associated with many enzymes, male and female fertility, protein synthesis, insulin production, skin integrity and many more processes.

- Iron necessary for the manufacture of red blood cells, cellular energy production and L-dopa metabolism.

- Specific minerals work in association with enzymes, activating them. They are known as "co-enzymes".

• Significant amounts of minerals are contained in dark green leafy vegetables, fish and seafood, nuts, seeds and dairy produce.

What does water do?

The body's largest component is water. Some of its functions include filtration by the kidneys, facilitation of good bowel movement, skin hydration and maintenance of mineral solution inside and between cells.

Conclusion

Adequate nutritional intake influences the healthy functioning of cells in the human body.

Note: It is noteworthy that in Parkinson's disease some minerals, although essential to cellular function, may be contraindicated. Laboratory tests to establish the nutritional status of each person is necessary for safe and best management.

Bibliography

■ Frank E. Berkowitz and Robert C. Jerris: Practical Medical Microbiology For Clinicians: 2016: WILEY Blackwell, US/Canada

■ Adrianne Bendich and Richard J. Deckelbaum: Preventive Nutrition, The Comprehensive Guide for Health Professionlsl Fifth Edition 2015: Humana Press/Springer International Publishing AG, Switzerland

■ Alan R Gaby: Nutritional Medicine: Second Edition 2017: Fritz Perlberg Publishing, US

■ Victor W. Rodwell, David A. Bender et al: 2015: Harper's Illustrated Biochemistry 30th Edition: McGraw Hill Education, USA: Protein Source p. 509

■ Sareen S. Gropper, Jack L. Smith, Timothy P. Carr: Advanced Nutrition and Metabolism Revised 7th Edition: Sengage Learning: 2017

Chapter 4

How the Brain Makes Dopamine
The Nutrition Connection!

SUMMARY

Dopamine is metabolized (transformed) by brain neurons (cells)
from dietary protein.
The transformation from food into the chemical messenger dopamine
is dependent on catalysts, known as enzymes.
These enzymes are also dependent on activators which are specific nutrients,
known as co-enzymes.

This entire metabolic process requires adequate cellular energy. Energy is
manufactured in the cells from specific nutrients in the diet and oxygen.

- In Parkinson's Disease, people are deficient in the neuro-transmitter (chemical messenger) known as dopamine. It controls movement and influences mood and stress response. Dopamine is metabolized (transformed) in the brain, its primary source from dietary protein[1].

- Specialised enzymes (enzymes make things happen), are activated by specific vitamins and minerals to assist in the step-by-step transformation of dietary protein into dopamine. These vitamins and minerals are known as co-enzymes or co-factors. They include zinc, vitamin B6, iron and tetrahydrobiopterin (folate derivative).

- Dopamine also influences the control of stress-related symptoms. Stress requires the body to produce adrenaline and the adrenal glands manufacture this hormone – *from dopamine*! The adrenal glands require vitamin B5 and vitamin C to maintain function. The enzyme which facilitates the transformation from dopamine to noradrenaline requires the co-enzymes vitamin C and copper. Methionine is needed by the enzyme which transforms noradrenaline (norepinephrine) to adrenaline (epinephrine).

- Cells need tremendous energy to make the transformation from dietary protein to dopamine! They produce energy during a special process known as the Citric Acid Cycle (Krebs Cycle). This process depends on glucose derived from food, as well as specific vitamins and minerals which include amongst other nutrients[2], vitamins B1, B2, B3, NADH, B5, C, Co-enzyme Q10, magnesium malate, iron, copper and fat. Biotin plays a vital role as a co-enzyme with acetyl co-enzyme A, in the final processing of food before it enters the energy cycle as glucose. Medium chain triglycerides (MCTs) in coconut oil offer an alternate fuel source, as glucose metabolism may be compromised in Parkinson's disease.

- Good bowel function and condition are necessary for the optimal absorption of nutrients and drugs.

Conclusion

It is obvious that in order for Parkinson's people to function as best as they are able, it is necessary to bring "nutritional awareness" into management programs. People who undergo "specialised" nutritional support of their biochemical individuality often report a better sense of well-being than those who do not.

- **See over page for further details and diagram** ➥

THE STEPS FROM DIETARY PROTEIN IN THE MOUTH TO...DOPAMINE IN THE BRAIN! ... & BEYOND!

1. After whole protein is eaten, such as EGGS, FISH, CHICKEN, SOY and TURKEY, digestion is initiated in the stomach by hydrochloric acid (involving zinc dependent carbonic anhydrase[3]). It is then further processed in the small bowel, by proteases.

2. After these processes, the digested protein is metabolized into tiny microscopic molecules called amino acids which are absorbed into the blood stream from the brush borders of the bowel. One of these amino acids is PHENYLALANINE.

   Phenylalanine metabolizes into another amino acid called TYROSINE.

3. In the blood stream, tyrosine transforms into L-DOPA and circulates up to the brain. The transformation from tyrosine to L-dopa is made possible by the action of the enzyme tyrosine hydroxylase, dependent on the co-enzymes iron[4] and tetrahydrobiopterin[5], itself dependent on NADH[6] (Vit. B3 derived).

4. The brain is protected by a special membrane called the Blood Brain Barrier (BBB), which protects the brain from unwanted and potentially dangerous substances.

   L-DOPA IS CARRIED THROUGH THIS BLOOD BRAIN BARRIER by a protein-like carrier and enters those specialised cells (neurons) in the brain, which are responsible for transforming it into DOPAMINE.

   The transformation, from L-dopa to dopamine, is made possible by the action of two enzymes. These are dopa decarboxylase, dependent on the co-enzyme vitamin B6[7], and catechol-o-methyltransferase (COMT).

5. Dopamine can be further metabolized into NORADRENALINE by the enzyme dopamine -hydroxylase, which is dependent on copper and vitamin C[8].

6. The enzyme phenylethanolamine N-methyltransferase which further metabolizes (converts) noradrenaline to ADRENALINE, requires the co-factor S-adenosylmethionine[9].

   The catecholemines noradrenaline (norepinephrine) and adrenaline (epinephrine) are used by the body to cope with different forms of stress.

DOPAMINE METABOLISM

DIETARY PROTEIN   (EGG, FISH, POULTRY, SOY)

– Hydrochloric acid, Carbonic anhydrase (zinc), Proteases

PHENYLALANINE

– Phenylalanine hydroxylase

TYROSINE

– Tyrosine hydroxylase (iron, tetrahydrobiopterin)

L-DOPA

– Catechol-o-methyltransferase (COMT), Dopa decarboxylase (vit B6)

DOPAMINE

– Dopamine -hydroxylase (copper, vit C)

NORADRENALINE

– Phenylethanolamine N-methyltransferase (S-adenosylmethionine)

ADRENALINE

The remit and scope of this book covers Protein to Dopamine and Adrenal Metabolism. Dopamine is metabolised further in the body. However, in people with Parkinson's Disease, it may be inefficiently processed but as yet its manipulation and support does not form part of the dynamic therapeutic spectrum.

References

1. Victor W. Rodwell, David A. Bender et al: 2015: Harper's Illustrated Biochemistry 30th Edition: McGraw Hill Education, USA: Protein Source p. 509
2. Victor W. Rodwell, David A. Bender et al: 2015: Harper's Illustrated Biochemistry 30th Edition: McGraw Hill Education, USA: p. 164
3. Sareen S. Gropper, Jack L. Smith, Timothy P. Carr: Advanced Nutrition and Metabolism Revised 7th Edition: Sengage Learning: 2017
4. Protein Sci: 1995: October 4: (10): pps. 2082-6
5. Victor L Davidson, Donald B Sittman: 1999: Biochemistry: Lippincott, Williams and Wilkins, Baltimore, Maryland, USA: p. 393
6. http://www.chem.qmul.ac.uk/iubmb/enzyme/reaction/misc/biopterin.html
7. Victor W. Rodwell, David A. Bender et al: 2015: Harper's Illustrated Biochemistry 30th Edition: McGraw Hill Education, USA: Protein Source p. 509
8. Victor W. Rodwell, David A. Bender et al: 2015: Harper's Illustrated Biochemistry 30th Edition: McGraw Hill Education, USA: Protein Source p. 510
9. Michael J Kuhar, Paster R Couceyro, Philip D. Lambert: 1999: American Soc. for Neurochemistry Basic Neurochemistry: Molecular Cellular and Medical Aspects Biosynthesis of Catacholemines 6th Edition

Chapter 5

Cellular Energy Production
Blood Sugar Regulation & Mood

People with Parkinson's Disease are often lacking in energy. This can be due to the disease itself, other ailments, the effects of medication,[1, 2] inadequate diet or stress. The metabolic ability of cells to generate adequate energy may be compromised.

Energy is made in the cells of the body during a special cycle known as the Citric Acid Cycle (or Krebs Cycle). To produce energy, cells use glucose, sourced from carbohydrates (fruit, vegetables, grains) together with specific vitamins and minerals also obtained from food. If the body does not have sufficient glucose from carbohydrates, it transforms protein and fats into glucose. In Parkinson's disease glucose metabolism may be a problem and medium chain triglycerides (MCTs) found in organic coconut oil can function as an alternative fuel source.

The many specific nutrients[3] needed in this energy-producing cycle include B vitamins, NADH, vitamin C, co-enzyme Q10, and the minerals iron and copper. Biotin is the essential co-enzyme with Acetyl CoA to metabolise carbohydrate and protein for entry into the energy cycle. The resulting miraculous energy is called adenosine-tri-phosphate (ATP) and is used by all the cells in the body to carry out their functions. Physical exercise increases oxygenation of cells, thereby enhancing energy production.

Stress influences and increases the concentration of glucose (blood sugar) in the blood. People with Parkinson's often note that stress exacerbates movement disturbance. This may be because adrenaline (epinephrine), released by the body during stress, is produced from dopamine – which has compromised production in those with Parkinson's Disease!

Specific nutritional management (appropriate food choices and intervals at which food is eaten), helps in the regulation of blood sugar levels. This in turn influences energy production, mood and concentration. A well- timed diet is helpful whether people are on dopaminergic medication or not. It has been demonstrated that low blood sugar (hypoglycaemia) affects brain energy and can damage neurones[4,5.] Blood sugar levels falling too low due to an inappropriate or irregular diet can result in tiredness, mood swings and anxiety.

Cautionary note

If energy levels, hunger, dizziness, inordinate amount of urination, lack of concentration and mood swings are a problem, these symptoms should urgently be reported to medical advisers.

Note for diabetics

Diabetic sufferers must always be advised by medical doctors, clinical nutritionists or dieticians. Each person has a different cellular biochemistry. The following nutritional facts may be considered: Insulin is complexed with zinc[6]. Chromium and vitamin B3 are involved in blood sugar regulation and are implicated in glucose tolerance factor (GTF).

How Energy and Blood Sugar Levels can be Supported

- Eating a small snack every two to three hours helps regulate blood sugar and energy levels. After four hours, glucose from the previous meal, has usually been absorbed. Snacks should contain a small portion of *complex carbohydrate* which breaks down into glucose more slowly and provides longer sustained energy. Glucose metabolism can be a problem in Parkinson's disease and medium chain triglycerides found in organic coconut oil are an alternative fuel source. Adequate exercise is important.

  ### Examples of recommended snacks:
  a) Gluten free crackers or bread, coconut oil spread and a little raw salad dressed with cold pressed olive or avocado oil or unrefined flaxseed oil

  b) Raw apple or cooked apple puree (complex carbohydrate) with a half a teaspoon of coconut oil.

  c) Soup with sweet potato (complex carbohydrate), other other green and orange coloured vegetables.

  Note: If L-dopa medication is not needed around this time, a little protein added to the snack may be helpful.

- Sugary food, refined carbohydrates, alcohol and caffeine should be gradually reduced. Substitute these with healthy delicious alternatives. Fruit juices should be diluted with still mineral or purified water.

- Oils, such as cold pressed olive or avocado oil or, unheated polyunsaturated oils, may slightly slow down glucose release and are suitable as food or salad dressings. Polyunsaturated oils must never be heated. Olive, coconut or avocado oil may be heated but not above 160°C as this will result in the production of trans fats.

Cellular Energy Production Blood Sugar Regulation & Mood

- Almonds and other nuts (not peanuts or cashews which may contain mycotoxins), together with fruit, are a good combination. Users of L-dopa need to be aware of the protein/L-dopa interaction (nuts contain a predominant amount of protein).

- If indicated medically, glucomannan fibre[7] can be taken as a supplement. This is a complex carbohydrate fibre, which is effective in stabilising blood sugar levels. However, the effects of this fibre on L-dopa ("Sinemet", "Madopar", "Stalevo" or equivalent drug) need to be assessed individually as the protein portion, although small, may compromise absorption of L-dopa.

- Nutritional biochemical tests assess the status of vitamins and minerals involved in the regulation of blood sugar. Chromium and vitamin B3 are implicated in glucose tolerance factor (GTF). Insulin and GTF are involved in blood sugar regulation. Deficiencies may need supplementing.

- Routine biochemical tests indicate diabetes or problems with glucose handling and insulin.

References

1. Werner P, Mytilineou C, Cohen G, Yahr MD: 1994: Impaired oxidation of pyruvate in human embryonic fibroblasts after exposure to L-dopa: pps. 157-62: European Journal of Pharmacology 263 (1-2)

2. Przedborski S, Jackson-Lewis V, Muthane U: 1993: Chronic levodopa administration alters cerebral mitochondrial respiratory chain activity: pps. 715-723: Ann Neurol: (34:5)

3. Bralley JA, Lord RS: Organic Acids in Urine: Laboratory Evaluations for Integrative and Functional Medicine: 2008: 2nd Edition: Metametrix Institute: 6:325

4. Wieloch T: 1985: Hypoglycemia-induced neuronal damage prevented by an N-methyl-D-aspartate antagonist: p. 681-3: Science: 230(4726)

5. Blaylock Russell L MD: 1997: Excitotoxins: pps.139, 156-158: Health Press, Santa Fe, New York, USA

6. Brody Tom: 1999: Nutritional Biochemistry: Second Edition: p. 808: Academic Press, New York, USA

7. Holford Patrick BSc Dip ION: 1992: Optimum Nutrition Workbook: p.148: ION Press, London, UK

Chapter 6

Biochemical Tests

Assessing patients on a cellular level enables healthcare professionals to plan patient management based on biochemical individuality. Some of the following tests may be useful tools in the assessment of metabolic, nutritional and general health status.

Comprehensive Haematology, Biochemistry and Ferritin – Blood (see Note 1)
General screens investigating immune function, response to infection, electrolytes, kidney function, liver function, haemoglobin, iron and lipid status.

Thyroid Function – Blood (see Note 2)
(TSH, FT4, FT3 Thyroid Antibodies)

Tyrosine metabolizes three ways – to form L-dopa, thyroxine and melanins.

Liver Detox Test (Phase 1, 2) – Saliva, Urine (see Note 3)
Phase 1 (Cytochrome P450) liver detoxification in patients with Parkinson's disease has been shown to be sub-optimal[1]. It is important to assess both phase 1 and phase 2 detoxification pathways in order to optimize nutritional management.

Toxic Metals / Pesticides Screens – Sweat / Blood (see Note 4) Patients may have been overly exposed to organophosphates and toxic metals, which affect neurones.

Minerals – Various screening methods (see Note 5)
Minerals are essential as co-enzymes. Examples: zinc in protein and essential fatty acid metabolism, magnesium in muscle relaxation and chromium is essential to glucose tolerance factor. Copper[2] is an essential coenzyme with dopamine β-hydroxylase and Vitamin C for adrenal metabolism. Manganese is a coenzyme with delta-6-desaturase and iron[3] essential for tyrosine hydroxylase and dopamine metabolism. Research indicates that routine administration of copper, iron and manganese may be contraindicated in Parkinson's disease management. Calcium may also be contraindicated because of an intracellular calcium block.

Magnesium (red cell) – Blood
Magnesium deficiency may contribute to muscle spasm and mitochondrial issues.

Fat Soluble Vitamins (Vitamin A, Carotenes, Vitamin E) – Blood (see Note 8)

Functional Tests
- Biotin – Blood (see Note 7)
  Coenzyme with Acetyl CoA, this is contributory to mitochondrial energy production.

- B Vitamins 1,2,6 – Blood (see Note 8)
  These are essential to the Citric Acid Cycle and the production of cellular energy (adenosine triphosphate, ATP). Vitamin B6 is the essential co-enzyme with dopa decarboxylase in the metabolic step from L-dopa to dopamine.

- Vitamin B3 – Blood (see note 8)
  Forms NADH for cell energy production and is a biopterin co-enzyme.

Vitamin B12 – (see Note 9)
This is associated with nervous/muscular function and appears to be required for tetrahydrobiopterin synthesis.

Folate – Blood (red blood cells, serum) (see Note 9)
Folate[4] is involved in the control of homocysteine and catecholemine (adrenaline and noradrenaline) synthesis and is linked with tetra-hydrobiopterin levels.

Methylation – (see Note 10)
Methylation is essential metabolism.

Digestive Enzymes – Various assessments (see Note 11)
Patients with Parkinson's disease may demonstrate deficiencies in the production of hydrochloric acid and/or pancreatic exocrine function. As dopamine is metabolized from protein it is essential that dietary protein be adequately digested to initiate this metabolic pathway. The digestion and absorption of carbohydrates and fats are essential to metabolism. Incompletely digested food molecules, particularly large protein molecules, may contribute to increased permeability of the gut mucosa.

Gut Permeability – Urine (see Note 12)

The integrity of the intestinal mucosa is essential for optimal nutritional absorption and protection against the entry of potential pathogens and allergens into the circulation. Permeability could be increased by disease, drugs, surgery, radiation and incompletely digested large protein molecules. Patients with increased gut permeability are often very fatigued.

Allergy (IgE) and Food Intolerances – Various methods of assessment

It has been observed clinically that certain foods and chemicals may aggravate symptoms in patients with Parkinson's Disease and general allergy and immune responses need to be taken into consideration.

Antioxidant Profile – Blood (see Note 13)

Oxidative stress is implicated in Parkinson's Disease.

Amino Acid Profile – Urine (see Note 14)

L-dopa is metabolized from dietary protein. It is useful to assess the general amino acid status of Parkinson's Disease patients.

Essential Fatty Acids – Blood (red blood cells) (see Note 15)

Essential Fatty Acids are essential to the nervous system, production of inflammatory and anti-inflammatory prostaglandins, skin integrity and produce ecosanoids.

Parasites – Stool, Blood, (see Note 16)

Parasites may be a problem for patients who present with chronic diarrhoea, fatigue, anal irritation and other symptoms.

Adrenal Stress Index – Saliva (see Note 17)

This test is a measure of cortisol and DHEA levels and is used as a bio- chemical marker of stress. Alteration of the levels of these hormones may have beneficial therapeutic effects.

Co-enzyme Q10 – Blood (serum) (see Note 15)

This nutrient plays a vital role in cell energy production and cardiovascular health.

Male / Female Hormones – Saliva and Blood (see Note 18)

Medical aspects - sexual, fertility, menstrual and menopausal problems.

Continued over page ➡

Metabolic Analysis Profile (Organic Acids) – Urine (see Note 19) Analysis of metabolic factors including the citric acid cycle (cell energy), neurotransmitter metabolites, markers of intestinal malabsorption and/or dysbiosis and co-factor dependent metabolites from amino acid catabolism

Superoxide Dismutase Detail Studies – Blood (See Note 20)

DNA Adducts – Blood (See Note 20)

Genetic-DNA Markers
Various tests to facilitate medical management

References

1. A Williams, S Sturman, G Steventon, R Waring: 1991: Metabolic Biomarkers of Parkinson's Disease – Acta Neurologica Scandinavica: Supplement 136: pps. 19-23

2. Jianyong Wang, , Mohammed F. Rahman et al: November 2009: NeuroToxicology Expression changes of dopaminergic system-related genes in PC12 cells induced by manganese, silver, or copper nanoparticles: Volume 30, Issue 6, , Pages 926–933

3. M. E. Götz, A. Freyberger, P. Riederer: 1990: Neurotransmitter Actions and Interactions: Oxidative stress: a role in the pathogenesis of Parkinson's disease: Volume 29 of the series Journal of Neural Transmission pps 241-249

4. Fernstrom JD: 2000: Am J Clin Nutr: 71(suppl): pps. 1669S-73S

Notes

1. Routine medical tests and some nutritional and allergy tests are carried out at general hospitals as well as at private medical laboratories, including The Doctors Laboratory, 55 Wimpole Street, London W1G 7DF Telephone: +44 (0)20 7460 4800. The laboratories listed below specialize in nutritional biochemistry.

2. Routine medical tests and some nutritional and allergy tests are carried out at general hospitals as well as at private medical laboratories, including The Doctors Laboratory, 55 Wimpole Street, London W1G 7DF Telephone: +44 (0)20 7460 4800. The laboratories listed below specialize in nutritional biochemistry.

3. Genova Diagnostics Europe, 356 West Barns Lane, New Malden, Surrey KT3 6NB UK: Telephone: +44 (0) 20 8336 7750 www.gdxuk.net

4. BioLab Medical Unit, 9 Weymouth Street, London, W1, UK: Telephone: +44 (0)20 7636 5959 Dr John McLaren-Howard

5. BioLab Medical Unit.

6. BioLab Medical Unit.

7. BioLab Medical Unit.

8. BioLab Medical Unit, 9 Weymouth Street, London, W1, UK Telephone: +44 (0)20 7636 5959

9. BioLab Medical Unit, 9 Weymouth Street, London, W1, UK Telephone: +44 (0)20 7636 5959

10. Regenerus Laboratories UK, +44 203 7500870 www.regeneruslabs.com,

11. Genova Diagnostics Europe, 356 West Barns Lane, New Malden, Surrey KT3 6NB UK: Telephone: +44 (0) 20 8336 7750 www.gdxuk.net

12. Genova Diagnostics Europe, 356 West Barns Lane, New Malden, Surrey KT3 6NB UK: Telephone: +44 (0) 20 8336 7750 www.gdxuk.net

13. BioLab Medical Unit, 9 Weymouth Street, London, W1, UK Telephone: +44 (0)20 7636 5959

14. Genova Diagnostics Europe, 356 West Barns Lane, New Malden, Surrey KT3 6NB UK: Telephone: +44 (0) 20 8336 7750 www.gdxuk.net

15. BioLab Medical Unit, 9 Weymouth Street, London, W1, UK Telephone: +44 (0)20 7636 5959

16. Regenerus Laboratories UK, +44 203 7500870 www.regeneruslabs.com,

17. Genova Diagnostics Europe, 356 West Barns Lane, New Malden, Surrey KT3 6NB UK: Telephone: +44 (0) 20 8336 7750 www.gdxuk.net

18. Genova Diagnostics Europe, 356 West Barns Lane, New Malden, Surrey KT3 6NB UK: Telephone: +44 (0) 20 8336 7750 www.gdxuk.net

19. Genova Diagnostics Europe, 356 West Barns Lane, New Malden, Surrey KT3 6NB UK: Telephone: +44 (0) 20 8336 7750 www.gdxuk.net

20. Acumen Laboratory, PO BOx 129, Tiverton, Devon EX16 OHA Telephone +44 (0) 7707 877175 email: acumen@hotmail.co.uk

Chapter 7

Nutritional Supplementation (Oral)

Between 1996 and 2016, each person with Parkinson's Disease seen at The London Pain Relief and Nutritional Support Clinic in London (aged between 16 and 75 years, males and females, some on L-dopa and others not) demonstrated deficiencies of various nutrients. These included vitamins, minerals and essential fatty acids. Some patients demonstrated deficiencies of digestive enzymes (hydrochloric acid and pancreatic enzymes). Permeability of the intestinal mucosa was often found to be increased. These results were obtained by using specialized medical laboratory tests.

They have demonstrated the necessity for personalised, nutritional supplementation as well as improved diet to optimize functional health. Support may include cell membrane integrity, methylation, anti-inflammatory prostaglandins and mitochondrial function. These aspects and others, including assessment of vitamin, mineral and essential fatty acid cellular status, pertinent in degenerative illness, require assessment and consideration for vital adjuvant care. Routine medical tests are also necessary.

In order to establish biochemical individuality for personalized medical and nutritional support, patients should undergo nutritional and routine medical laboratory tests. Diet change and nutritional supplementation should always be under the guidance of a nutritionist or doctor. Nutritional supplements do affect body biochemistry and there can be interactions between nutrients and drugs. **Biochemical individuality is an essential consideration in nutritional and medical support.**

However, nutritional deficiencies also occur in people who do not have Parkinson's disease and their impoverished cellular environment will equally require support.

Supplements designed to be taken sublingually (under the tongue) or transdermally, if available, are more easily absorbed than capsules and tablets in people with absorption problems. However, if absorption remains a problem after oral nutritional therapy, patients may benefit from intravenous nutritional support.

Following is a list of commonly used nutritional supplements. Their use should routinely be based on patients' biochemical individuality, always administered under professional supervision. There may be serious contraindications to taking some in individual cases.[1a]

- **Vitamin A** (Vitamin A and Carotenes must never be taken without medical supervision)
Implicated, amongst other functions, in the integrity of the gut mucosa and is an important antioxidant. Vitamin A and carotenes should only be administered in small doses, only if medically indicated. **There may be serious health contraindications.**

- **Vitamin B Complex** (Methyl B Complex to assist methylation)
B vitamins are best taken as a complex. The suggested dose is approximately 25mg daily for each, but a higher dose of vitamin B5 for adrenal support. B vitamins play a role in mitochondrial energy production. Most L-dopa drugs contain a decarboxylase inhibitor, which prevents the breakdown of L-dopa before entering the brain. As such, vitamin B6 can be part of nutritional support for patients taking "Sinemet"[1b]/Stalevo/ "Madopar"[2]. It is an essential co-enzyme in the metabolic step between L-dopa and dopamine[3,4].

- **NADH** (Vitamin B3 derivative)
This may stimulate L-dopa biosynthesis[5], is the co-factor for the enzyme which forms tetrahydrobiopterin and is involved in cell energy metabolism[6].

- **Vitamin B12**
This is implicated in neuromuscular function, methylation (methylcobalamine) and appears to be required for tetrahydrobiopterin synthesis.

- **Vitamin C** (monitoring needed if patients on anticoagulant therapy)
This is a co-enzyme with dopamine ß hydroxylase and influences platelet aggregation (clumping of blood cells).

- **Vitamin D3**
Deficiencies have been detected in Parkinson's Disease[7,7a]. It is implicated in bone metabolism.

- **Iron – possible contraindications (oxidative stress) with Parkinson's disease**
Iron supplements should be taken at least two hours away from L-dopa administration and two hours away from taking zinc. Iron is best absorbed together with vitamin C. Although it is the essential co-enzyme for metabolism of levodopa and red blood cells, it should only be taken *if deficient and strictly medically monitored.*

- Zinc
  This is implicated in many enzyme functions, protein metabolism and repair mechanisms. It should be administered at least 2 hours away from iron. (see Note 1 on page 24). Dosage should be prudent.

- Magnesium
  Deficiency can exacerbate muscle spasm and it is a co-enzyme in fatty acid and energy metabolism.

- Calcium – possible contraindications (intracellular calcium block) in Parkinson's disease
  It is best absorbed in the citrate or amino acid chelate form and is part of the bone matrix. However, for bone integrity, vitamin D3 and magnesium are also essential, as well as weight bearing exercise. These considerations are essential if calcium administration is contraindicated with the intracellular calcium problem.

- Electrolytes
  Electrolyte combinations include sodium, potassium, calcium, magnesium and chloride amongst others and are prescribed by the attendant physician when clinically indicated for example for dehydration.

- Manganese – may be contraindicated in Parkinson's disease
  This is an important co-enzyme with delta-6-desaturase fatty acid metabolism, which produces anti-inflammatory prostaglandins.

- Chromium
  This is implicated in blood sugar control.

- Broad-spectrum Amino Acids / Poly-peptides
  These forms of pre-digested protein are for anabolic (building blocks for the body) function. Pre-digested amino acids and poly-peptides are more quickly absorbed than protein food, which makes them eminently suitable for those who need L-dopa medication at shorter intervals. Protein supplementation may be necessary if patients are on a reduced protein diet or suffering from mal-absorption or loss of muscle mass.

- Gingko biloba
  This is an anti-oxidant which dilates capillaries and improves circulation.

- Anti-oxidants[8, 9, 10, 11, 12]
  These are implicated in control of free-radicals and include alpha lipoic acid,[12] vitamins C and E as well as selenium, zinc and glutathione (reduced form or as the pre-curser n-acetyl cysteine (low doses as may act as an excitotoxin)).

- **N-acetyl-cysteine[13](Glutathione Precursor)**
  This stimulates the body's own production of glutathione[14] which is an antioxidant and also involved in the liver detoxification process. However, in large doses it can act as an excitotoxin. Some practitioners prefer to give glutathione intravenously.

- **Acetyl-L-carnitine[15]**
  Acetyl-L-carnitine is an important antioxidant.

- **Butyric Acid**
  Butyric acid is an agent for repair of the intestinal mucosa, when gut permeability is increased. It is a short chain fatty acid and occurs naturally in the gastro-intestinal tract of humans. It is a by-product of the fermentation of fibre by lactic bacteria, such as Lactobacillus acidophilus. Butyric acid should not be confused with gamma amino butyric acid (GABA), which is an amino acid.

  Note: glutamine is often prescribed for repair of the intestinal mucosa. However, in therapeutic doses it is contra-indicated in Parkinson's Disease as it may manifest as an excitotoxin. Butyric acid also contributes to membrane integrity and can be used as a substitute.

- **Phosphatidyl choline[16]**
  This is for cell membrane stability.

- **Essential fatty acids (Omega 6 and Omega 3)[17]**
  These enhance cellular membrane integrity, upregulate the immune system and are involved in the metabolization of anti- inflammatory and inflammatory prostaglandins series 1, 2 and 3. Omega 6 is found in primrose and borage oils, Omega 3 in fish oils and arachadonic acid in saturated fat.

- **Methyl Folate[18]** is involved in the control of homocysteine and catecholamine synthesis. It has been linked with tetrahydro- biopterin[19] levels. Methyl folate is implicated in methylation.

- **Digestive enzymes**
  Hydrochloric acid and pancreatic enzymes can be prescribed if deficiencies are medically demonstrated.

- **Probiotics**
  These include Lactobacillus GG / longum / plantarum / rhamnosus / salivarius / acidophilus, bulgaricus, Bifidobacterium bifidum and other cultures of intestinal bacteria[20]. *Each may have its individual indication and contraindication.* Gut immunity may be enhanced by these friendly cultures

of intestinal bacteria. Probiotics and saccharomyces boulardi need to be supplemented alongside antibiotic therapy. Prebiotics (nutrition for probiotics), such as fructo- oligosaccharides and galacto-oligosaccharides, may sometimes be indicated. Brain – derived neurotrophic factor (BDNF) may be enhanced by probiotics, thus positively influencing dopamine metabolism.[21] Alternating diverse strains of probiotics is recommended.

- **Co-enzyme Q10**
  This nutrient plays a role in cell energy production[22]. It is also important in cardiovascular health[23].

- **Biotin**
  Biotin is the important co-enzyme with Acetyl CoA for gluconeogenesis and energy production.[24]

  NOTE: It is interesting to note the significant zinc deficiency in patients whether they take L-dopa or not. Significant zinc deficiency in the cerebrospinal fluid of Parkinson's Disease patients has been demonstrated in a controlled trial[25]. Zinc was also deficient in another controlled study assessing the nutritional status of patients with Parkinson's Disease[26].

- **Curcumin (Curcuma longa)**
  Curcumin exhibits antioxidant, anti-inflammatory properties, crosses the blood-brain barrier and is neuroprotective in neurological disorders. Several studies in different experimental models of PD strongly support the clinical application of curcumin in PD[27].

References

1a. Powers K M, Smith-Weller T et all: June 10, 2003: Neurology, Vol 60, No 11, Parkinson's Disease Risks Asscociated With Dietary Iron, Mangonese and other nutrient intakes: pps 1761-1766

1b. ABPI Compendium of Data Sheets and Summaries of Product Characteristics (1999-2000): Datapharm Publications Limited, London, UK: p. 371

2. Ibid: p. 1334

3. Dr Geoffrey Leader MB ChB FRCA and Lucille Leader Dip ION: 1996: Parkinson's Disease - The New Nutritional Handbook: Denor Press, London, UK: p.6

4. J Hywel Thomas PhD FIBiol and B Gillham PhD: 1989:Wills' Biochemical Basis of Medicine: Butterworth Heinemann: Oxford, UK: p.417

5. Volc D, Birkmayer JG, Vrecki C, Birkmayer W: 1993: NADH - A new therapeutic approach to Parkinson's Disease. Comparison of oral and parenteral application: Acta Neurologica Scandinavica Suppl. 146: pps. 32-35

6. Nadlinger K, Westerthaler W, Storga-Tomic D, Birkmayer J.G.D: Extracellular metabolisation of NADH by blood cells correlates with intracellular ATP levels: November 2002: Biochimica et Biophysica Acta (BBA)/General Subjects: Volume 1573, Number 2, 14: pps. 177-182

7. Y Sato, M Kikyuama, K Oizumi: 1997: High Prevalance of Vitamin D deficiency and reduced bone mass in Parkinson's Disease: Neurology 49(5): pps. 1273-79

7a Khanh vinh quõc Luong, Lan Thi Hoàng Nguyên: December 2012: Journal of Neuroscience Research: Vol 90 Issue 12: Vit D in Parkinson Disease: pps. 2227-2236

8. European Journal of Pharmacology 263 (1-2): 1994: September 22: Impaired oxidation of pyruvate in human embryonic fibroblasts after exposure to Ldopa: pps.157-62

9. C W Olanow: 1989: Attempts to obtain neuroprotection in Parkinson's Disease: Neurology 49: Supplement 1: S26-S33

10. Pong K: 2003: Oxidative stress in neurodegenerative diseases, therapeutic implications for superoxide dismutase mimetics: Expert Opinion on Biological Therapy: 3: pps. 127-39

11. Juurlin H, Paterson PG: 1998: Review of oxidative stress in brain and spinal cord injury, Suggestions for pharmacological and nutritional management strategies: B: J Spinal Cord Med Oct: 21 (4): pps. 309-334

12. Dr David Perlmutter MD: 2000: BrainRecovery.Com: Perlmutter Health Center, Naples, FL, USA: p25

13. Ibid: p. 26

14. Oja SS, Jankay R, Varga V, Saransaari P: 2000: Modulation of Glutamate Receptor Functions by Glutathione: Neurochem Int Aug-Sept 37 (2-3): pps. 299-306

15. Steffen V et al: 1995: Effect of Intraventricular injection of l-methyl-4- phenylpyridinium protection by acetyl-L-carnitine: Human Exp Toxicol: (14): pps. 865-871

16. Cui Z, Houweling M, Review: 2002: Phosphatidyl choline and Cell Death: Biochemica et Biophysica Acta: 1585:pps.87-96

17. Yehuda S,Rabinovitz S et al: 1998: Review: Fatty Acids and Brain Peptides: Peptides: Vol 19. No 2: pps. 407-419

18. Fernstrom JD: 2000: Am J Clin Nutr: 71(suppl): pps. 1669 S-73S

19. Hamon CG et al: 1986: The Effect of Tetrahydrofolate on Tetrahydrobiopterin Metabolism: J Ment Defic Res 30: pps. 179-183

20. Leon Chaitow ND DO and Natasha Trenev: 1990: Probiotics: Thorsons: An Imprint of HarperCollins Publishers, London, UK : pps. 24-25

21. Berton et al: 2006: Nature Reviews Neuroscience 7:pps.137-151

22. Shults C et al: 1999: A Possible Role of Co-enzyme Q10 in the Etiology and Treatment of Parkinson's Disease: BioFactors (2-4): pps. 267 - 272

23. Langsjoen H, Langsjoen P et al: 1994: Usefulness of Co-enzyme Q10 in Clinical Cardiology: A Long Term Study: Mol. Aspects Med: 15 Suppl. S165-S175

24. Victor Davidson, Donald Sittman: 1999: Biochemistry: Lippencott, Williams, Wilkins USA: p328

25. Ward NI et al: 1988: Trace Element Status of Cerebrospinal Fluid of Individuals with Neurological Diseases by ICP-MS Trace Elements Analysis in Diagnosis and Pathological States: Vol 5: Proceedings of the 5th International Workshop in Nuremburg, Rep of Germany: Trace Element Analytical Chemistry in Medicine and Biology: Walter de Gruyter & Co, Germany / USA: pps. 513-550

26. Abbot RA et al: 1992: A Diet, Body Size and Micronutrient Status in Parkinson's Disease: European Journal of Clinical Nutrition 46(12): pps. 879 – 884

27. B. Mythri, R.; M. Srinivas Bharath, M. Current Pharmaceutical Design, Volume 18, Number 1, January 2012, pp. 91-99(9): Bentham Science Publishers

Bibliography

■ Victor W. Rodwell, David A. Bender et al: 2015: Harper's Illustrated Biochemistry 30th Edition: McGraw Hill Education, USA: Protein Source

■ Victor W. Rodwell, David A. Bender et al: 2015: Harper's Illustrated Biochemistry 30th Edition: McGraw Hill Education, USA:

■ Sareen S. Gropper, Jack L. Smith, Timothy P. Carr: Advanced Nutrition and Metabolism. Revised 7th Edition: Sengage Learning: 2017

■ Alan R. Gaby:2017:Nutritional Medicine,Second Edition: Fritz Perlberg Publishing Concord NH

■ The Encyclopedia of Natural Medicine Third Edition Paperback – 20 Nov 2014 by Michael T. Murray M.D. (Author), Joseph Pizzorno (Author)

■ Protein Sci: 1995: October 4: (10):

■ Victor L Davidson, Donald B Sittman: 1999: Biochemistry: Lippincott, Williams and Wilkins, Baltimore, Maryland, USA:

■ http://www.chem.qmul.ac.uk/iubmb/enzyme/reaction/misc/biopterin.html

■ Victor W. Rodwell, David A. Bender et al: 2015: Harper's Illustrated Biochemistry 30th Edition: McGraw Hill Education, USA: Protein Source

■ Victor W. Rodwell, David A. Bender et al: 2015: Harper's Illustrated Biochemistry 30th Edition: McGraw Hill Education, USA: Protein Source

■ Michael J Kuhar, Paster R Couceyro, Philip D. Lambert: 1999: American Soc. for Neurochemistry Basic Neurochemistry: Molecular Cellular and Medical Aspects Biosynthesis of Catacholemines 6th Edition

■ Michael Ash: 2008: Atypical Depression, The Immune System, Probiotics and Clinical Application:The Stressed Gut-The Stressed Brain: Royal Society of Medicine Presentation: Food and Health Forum: London UK

Chapter 8

Improving Bowel Function

The authors cannot be held responsible for individual medical problems associated with bowel dysfunction and the recommendations made must be approved by patients' medical advisors.

Hippocrates, the father of modern medicine, made the famous recommendation: *"Make food your medicine".*

In the case of bowel function, this could indeed be helpful!

Both constipation, incontinence and diarrhoea can be a problem in Parkinson's Disease. The reasons for these difficulties must be assessed by the medical profession. However, if the causes are purely functional, without any specific pathology (disease), the following protocols can be helpful. It is important, however, for patients to urgently alert their medical practitioners if symptoms do not improve. If there is any pain and distension accompanying lack of bowel movement, this may signify bowel obstruction, which needs immediate medical intervention.

Diarrhoea
This may be caused by reaction to drugs, Inflammatory Bowel Disease (IBD), The Irritable Bowel Syndrome (IBS), parasites, bowel cancer or other diseases. If disease has been ruled out and drugs reviewed, the following recommendations may be helpful:

a)   Sufficient filtered or still mineral water, drunk over the day, to replace loss of fluid. The doctor should be approached for a possible prescription for "electrolytes" as these may be lost as a consequence of diarrhoea or vomiting.

b)   The stool may be bound with apple pectin[1]. Apple pectin slows down the transit time of food through the bowel. This is available as a nutritional supplement in either powder or tablet / capsule form. Taking probiotics may be helpful.

c)   Anti-diarrhoeal drugs may need to be medically prescribed and response medically monitored.

Constipation

a) 8–10 glasses of filtered or still mineral water should be drunk over the day.

b) Some fibrous foods are helpful. Seemingly effective seems to be prunes (soaked in boiling water to rehydrate) or figs (rehydrated if dried). It is not sufficient to take one serving only per day. Prunes and figs should be taken in small quantities (2-3 pieces) between meals *spread at intervals over the whole day.*

   However, wheat-based fibre is not appropriate for PD sufferers. Wheat contains gluten, a dense protein, which may interfere with the absorption of L-dopa medication[2]. It also contains gliadin which may be contra-indicated in neurological conditions. Research has demonstrated that wheat germ may cause increased intestinal permeability[3], which is not desirable.

c) Cabbage, lettuce, carrots and radishes are beneficial as these readily absorb moisture[4].

d) Fruit, especially melons and plums, are best eaten between meals to reduce feelings of bloating and flatulence.

e) Take a glass of still filtered water or coconut water several minutes before each meal. Ensure at least 9-10 glasses of fluid spread over the day. Coconut water contains potassium which is helpful to intestinal function. Starting the day with a glass of warm water may be helpful.

f) Probiotics ("friendly" gut bacteria) include Lactobacillus plantarum/ rhamnosus / salivarius, Bifidobacterium bifidum, Lactobacillus acidophilus, Lactobacillus bulgaricus and other cultures of intestinal bacteria. Gut immunity is enhanced by these and other friendly cultures of intestinal bacteria. Probiotics should be refrigerated and need to be supplemented if patients have taken antibiotics. Saccharomyces boulardi is also recommended when taking antibiotics. Prebiotics (small doses), such as fructooligosaccharides, can sometimes help with constipation. Professional advice is always necessary.

g) Regular exercise and specialised abdominal massage can be helpful.

h) Osteopathic assessment and gentle manipulation may sometimes be indicated.

i) Patients should make the time to sit regularly on the toilet, 10 to 20 minutes after each meal, even if there is no urge to defecate in order to train a gastro-colic reflex. They should sit and relax for at least 10 minutes without straining or pushing. It is hoped that eventually a rhythm for bowel emptying will establish itself[5]

j) Patients should not delay going to the toilet at any time when they do feel the urge to defecate.

k) Occasionally a gentle enema may be indicated. This need must be assessed and supervised by the medical practitioner.

l) Harsh laxatives containing senna and cascara are contraindicated for regular use. They can cause melanosis in the intestinal tract and eventually inhibit spontaneous function of the bowel.

m) Phillips Milk of Magnesia can be helpful after a day of no bowel movement.

It is important, however, to consult a medical practitioner urgently when there is no bowel movement, together with distension and pain, in spite of laxative supplementation. This could be an indication of bowel obstruction.

n) Medically supervised use of products containing magnesium such as Kirkman Buffered Magnesium Oxide and Caricol (papaya concentrate) a stool facilitator. These products may be used routinely as they do not cause problems associated with melanosis and do not inhibit spontaneous bowel function as do chronic use of strong laxatives. In some cases a suppository may be prescribed to facilitate the initial passing of stool or Lactulose to soften the stool. Medical monitoring of response is always necessary.

Neurogastroenterology
Persistent intestinal problems associated with constipation, diarrhoea and incontinence may benefit from referral to a Neurogastroenterology unit.

References
1. Heaton KW: 1991: Fibre and Bulk Preparations: Extract from Gastrointestinal Transit (Pathophysiology and Pharmacology): Wrightson Biomedical Publishing Ltd, UK: pps. 212, 213
2. Kempster P A MD MRCP FRACP, M C Wahlqvist MD FRACP: 1994: Dietary factors in the management of Parkinson's Disease: Nutrition Reviews Vol 52, No. 2
3. Pusztai A: 1993: Dietary lectins are metabolic signals for the gut and modulate immune and hormone functions: European Journal Clin Nutr 47: pps. 691-99
4. Kaman Betty PhD: 1991: New Facts About Fibre: Nutrition Encounter Inc: Novato, California, USA: pps. 19, 59
5. Trattler Ross ND DO: 1987: Better Health through Natural Healing: Thorsons Publishers Limited: London, UK: p. 191

Chapter 9

At what Intervals should L–Dopa be taken Orally?
Monitoring Schemes for a Smoother "ON–OFF" Period

The following personalised drug response assessment schemes are exclusive to the integrated medical and nutritional work of the authors. They are based on clinical assessment of individual patients. Patients are advised to consult their medical advisors before embarking on any assessment scheme and then again with their results. The authors cannot take responsibility for the individual results and drug applications by readers. It must always be remembered that due to the fluctuating nature of Parkinson's disease, the results are not always predictable.

In order to assess how long your L-dopa medication lasts for you, carry out the following short monitoring schemes over a few days. Fill in the tables provided for each assessment. The results will serve as an invaluable guide for you and your doctors to assess how long your L-dopa works for you and what the minimum dose is that will effectively serve you.

Carry out each trial, noting: (see pages 34 – 45)

- The dose of L-dopa, or L-dopa with other anti-Parkinson drugs

- The time taken for "kick-in" (the time taken to establish effect)

- The length of time L-dopa is effective

- Only eat the prescribed foods (after your L-dopa has "kicked in"), as these will not compromise the absorption of L-dopa. It is essential to eat immediately the drug has taken effect.

- After the morning's trial is completed, continue with your normal regime (drugs and food) for the rest of the day. *Regard the drugs on the monitoring trial as in place of your usual first prescription of the day.*

At the end of each day's monitoring scheme, you will be able to assess how often you need to take L-dopa

To assist in estimating this, take note of the following examples:

Examples

a) If your "standard" dose of L-dopa lasts for 3½ hours and it has taken ½ hour to "kick-in", you may need to take L-dopa approximately every 3 hours. Taking L-dopa medication ½ hour before the time that it is likely to wear off could help to smooth out and reduce the "on-off" discomfort.

b) If you notice that your "standard" dose of L-dopa lasts for 4 hours and it has taken 45 minutes to "kick in", you may need to take L-dopa approximately every 3¼ hours. Taking L-dopa medication
45 minutes before the time that it is likely to wear off could help to smooth out and reduce the "on-off" discomfort.

However, if taking your L-dopa doses according to the above scheme (in order to smooth out the "on-off" period) increases your usual amount of milligrams prescribed per day OR increases your movement disturbance, you must urgently review your drug regime with your neurologist. Your specialist may wish to prescribe smaller doses of L-dopa, enabling you to take it more frequently.

Professor Aroldo Rossi, of The Department of Neurology and Psychiatry at the University of Perugia, Italy, recommends that L-dopa be introduced at a low dosage and then escalated very slowly, if required.

Oral "controlled release[1]" L-dopa preparations are not used in our monitoring schemes as they are not as predictable as the "standard" formulae. However, they do have their place in the general therapeutic spectrum, especially at night, when there is no need for dietary flexibility. Nonetheless Duodopa, a controlled-release L-dopa preparation that is administered by tube directly into the duodenum, is used during the day (see page 49), [but not in these monitoring schemes].

Continued over page ➥

31

ASSESSMENT SCHEMES

Choose the section which is relevant to your personal drug regime. However, it is usually helpful to begin monitoring responses with the smallest dose of L-dopa ('Madopar', 'Sinemet', 'Stalevo').

Only one assessment should be performed per day. The first assessment should be a) of the relevant section and if possible, all the variants of that assessment scheme should be carried out.

Note: it is perfectly acceptable to leave an interval of any length between assessments.

1. **L–dopa includes Decarboxylase Inhibitors**
   a) "Madopar" 50/12.5 mg / "Sinemet" 12.5/50 mg
   b) "Madopar" 50/12.5 mg / "Sinemet" 12.5/50 mg plus COMT Inhibitor
   c) "Madopar" 50/12.5 mg / "Sinemet" 12.5/50 mg plus Agonist
   d) "Madopar" 50/12.5 mg / "Sinemet" 12.5/50 mg plus COMT Inhibitor
       plus Agonist

2. **L–dopa includes Decarboxylase Inhibitors**
   a) "Madopar" 100/25 mg / "Sinemet" 25/100 mg
   b) "Madopar" 100/25 mg / "Sinemet" 25/100 mg plus COMT Inhibitor
   c) "Madopar" 100/25 mg / "Sinemet" 25/100 mg plus Agonist
   d) "Madopar" 100/25 mg / "Sinemet" 25/100 mg plus COMT Inhibitor
       plus Agonist

3. **L–dopa includes Decarboxylase Inhibitor and COMT Inhibitor**
   a) "Stalevo" 50/12.5/200 mg
   b) "Stalevo" 50/12.5/200 mg plus Agonist
   c) "Stalevo" 100/25/200 mg
   d) "Stalevo" 100/25/200 mg plus Agonist
   e) "Stalevo" 200/50/200 mg
   f) "Stalevo" 200/50/200 mg plus Agonist

Note:
The Decarboxylase Inhibitors include Benserazide Hydrochloride and Anhydrous Carbidopa. Entacapone is the COMT Inhibitor.

Other anti-Parkinson drugs, including MAO Type B Inhibitors ('Zelapar', 'Azilect'), may be added sequentially to any of the above monitoring schemes.

Glossary

L-dopa
This is the synthetic pharmaceutical medication which replaces the natural substance normally produced in cells but which is reduced in Parkinson's patients. It is metabolized (converted) to the neuro- transmitter dopamine, in the brain. L-dopa is also found in the mucuna pruriens bean and dosage has been standardised pharmaceutically by a specific company.

Dopa decarboxylase inhibitor (benserazide in "Madopar" and carbidopa in "Sinemet" and "Stalevo")
This is added to L-dopa drugs in order to inhibit L-dopa metabolizing to dopamine before it needs to cross the Blood Brain Barrier. This enables vitamin B6 (the co-enzyme which facilitates the transformation from L-dopa to dopamine), to be given.

COMT Inhibitor
Levodopa (L-dopa) is mainly metabolized (processed) by the enzymes dopa decarboxylase and catechol-O-methyltransferase (COMT). When L-dopa is administered with a peripheral dopa decarboxylase inhibitor, such as benserazide or carbidopa, levodopa metabolism with COMT increases, resulting in increased production of 3-O-methyldopa. This metabolite competes with L-dopa for transport across the blood-brain barrier and may decrease the absorption and efficacy of levodopa in the brain[2,3.] A COMT Inhibitor prevents the over-production of 3-O-methyldopa, enabling more L-dopa to be available for transport across the Blood Brain Barrier. In summary for non-scientific readers, COMT Inhibitors will improve the absorption of L-dopa medication.

Agonist
A drug, which upon binding to a receptor on the pre or post-synaptic membrane, produces a response similar to that caused by the neurotransmitter released at the synapse. This is because Agonists are structurally similar to dopamine, meaning they can simulate its action.

Monoamine Oxidase Type B (MAO-B) Inhibitor
The enzyme, Monoamine OxidaseType B, is implicated in the catabolism (breakdown) of dopamine. Inhibition of this oxidative process can be helpful in Parkinson's Disease.

Continued over page ❖

SCHEME 1(a) HOW LONG AM I "ON": with L-dopa Madopar 50mg/12.5mg or Sinemet 12.5mg/50mg (also applies to Zandopa HP200)?

IMPORTANT NOTE
Your L-dopa medication will not serve you optimally if:
- you are stressed in any way during the period of this test
- you have a difficult bowel movement
- you are not well (apart from Parkinson's)
- you eat foods which are not on the list below

If any of these conditions apply, redo the test on another day when you have no extra stress or ailments.

Instruction	Time / Description
Do not take L-dopa for 7 hours before starting this trial	
1. Wake up in the morning: do not eat or drink but you **can** have a glass of water. Describe symptoms as you awake (e.g. tremor, stiffness, etc). Take one dose of standard L-dopa (NOT CONTROLLED RELEASE). Do not eat with L-dopa. Note the time. Have some dilute apple juice after 10 minutes. Eat Breakfast as soon as the drug takes effect. If you do not have any symptoms as yet, wait until you do before taking L-dopa as per the above instruction. Whilst waiting, eat only fruit (no citrus) and drink herb tea.	Symptoms: L-dopa time:
2. Write the time of relief of symptoms. Only eat after the drug has taken effect ("kicked in").	"Kick-in" time:
3. Write the time of breakfast (see the **specific** breakfast menu below)	Breakfast time:
4. Write the time of the **beginning** of "wear-off" of L-dopa.	Beginning "wear-off" time:
5. Write the time of bowel movement. Describe (difficult / normal).	Time: Difficult/normal

THE SPECIFIC BREAKFAST ON THE EXPERIMENTAL DAY
Eat only the following specific foods at breakfast, immediately after your L-dopa has kicked in. These will not compromise absorption of L-dopa[10,11].

Banana, millet cereal (no other grains added) with water. Cereal can be sweetened with jam or fruit (no citrus). Peppermint or camomile tea. Alternatively, eat vegetable soup (sweet potato, leeks, courgettes, parsley), fruit (no citrus), mint tea.

Resume your usual food and drug regime after completing this trial.

These L-dopa doses on the trial replace your usual first doses of the day.

SCHEME 1(b) **HOW LONG AM I "ON": with L-dopa Madopar 50mg/12.5mg or Sinemet 12.5mg/50mg plus COMT Inhibitor?**

IMPORTANT NOTE

Your L-dopa medication will not serve you optimally if:

■ you are stressed in any way during the period of this test
■ you have a difficult bowel movement
■ you are not well (apart from Parkinson's)
■ you eat foods which are not on the list below

If any of these conditions apply, redo the test on another day when you have no extra stress or ailments.

Instruction	Time / Description
Do not take dopaminergic drugs for 7 hours before starting this trial	
1. Wake up in the morning: do not eat or drink but you **can** have a glass of water. Describe symptoms as you awake (e.g. tremor, stiffness, etc). Take one dose of standard L-dopa (NOT CONTROLLED RELEASE). Do not eat with L-dopa. Note the time you take L-dopa and COMT inhibitor. Have some dilute apple juice after 10 minutes. Eat Breakfast as soon as the drug takes effect. If you do not have any symptoms as yet, wait until you do before taking L-dopa as per the above instruction. Whilst waiting, eat only fruit (no citrus) and drink herb tea.	Symptoms: L-dopa & COMT Inhibitor time:
2. Write the time of relief of symptoms. Only eat after the drug has taken effect ("kicked in").	"Kick-in" time:
3. Write the time of breakfast (see the **specific** breakfast menu below)	Breakfast time:
4. Write the time of the **beginning** of "wear-off " of L-dopa.	Beginning "wear-off " time:
5. Write the time of bowel movement. Describe (difficult / normal).	Time: Difficult/normal

THE SPECIFIC BREAKFAST ON THE EXPERIMENTAL DAY

Eat only the following specific foods at breakfast, immediately after your L-dopa has kicked in. These will not compromise absorption of L-dopa[10,11].

Banana, millet cereal (no other grains added) with water. Cereal can be sweetened with jam or fruit (no citrus). Peppermint or camomile tea. Alternatively, eat vegetable soup (sweet potato, leeks, courgettes, parsley), fruit (no citrus), mint tea.

Resume your usual food and drug regime after completing this trial.
These L-dopa doses on the trial replace your usual first doses of the day.

SCHEME 1(c) HOW LONG AM I "ON": with L-dopa Madopar 50mg/12.5mg or Sinemet 12.5mg/50mg plus Agonist?

IMPORTANT NOTE
Your L-dopa medication will not serve you optimally if:

- you are stressed in any way during the period of this test
- you have a difficult bowel movement
- you are not well (apart from Parkinson's)
- you eat foods which are not on the list below

If any of these conditions apply, redo the test on another day when you have no extra stress or ailments.

Instruction	Time / Description
Do not take dopaminergic drugs for 7 hours before starting this trial	
1. Wake up in the morning: do not eat or drink but you **can** have a glass of water. Describe symptoms as you awake (e.g. tremor, stiffness, etc). Take one dose of standard L-dopa (NOT CONTROLLED RELEASE). Do not eat with L-dopa. Note the time. Have some dilute apple juice after 10 minutes. Eat Breakfast as soon as the drug takes effect. If you do not have any symptoms as yet, wait until you do before taking L-dopa as per the above instruction. Whilst waiting, eat only fruit (no citrus) and drink herb tea.	Symptoms: L-dopa time:
2. Write the time of relief of symptoms. Only eat after the drug has taken effect ("kicked in").	"Kick-in" time:
3. Write the time of breakfast (see the specific breakfast menu below) and take the Agonist with a glass of still mineral or purified water. If nausea is a problem, take the Agonist at the end of the meal.	Breakfast time:
4. Write the time of the ***beginning*** of "wear-off " of L-dopa.	Beginning "wear-off " time:
5. Write the time of bowel movement. Describe (difficult / normal).	Time: Difficult/normal

THE SPECIFIC BREAKFAST ON THE EXPERIMENTAL DAY
Eat only the following specific foods at breakfast, immediately after your L-dopa has kicked in. These will not compromise absorption of L-dopa10,11.

Banana, millet cereal (no other grains added) with water. Cereal can be sweetened with jam or fruit (no citrus). Peppermint or camomile tea. Alternatively, eat vegetable soup (sweet potato, leeks, courgettes, parsley), fruit (no citrus), mint tea.

Resume your usual food and drug regime after completing this trial.
These L-dopa doses on the trial replace your usual first doses of the day.

SCHEME 1(d) HOW LONG AM I "ON": with L-dopa Madopar 50mg/12.5mg or Sinemet 12.5mg/50mg plus COMT Inhibitor plus Agonist?

IMPORTANT NOTE
Your L-dopa medication will not serve you optimally if:
- you are stressed in any way during the period of this test
- you have a difficult bowel movement
- you are not well (apart from Parkinson's)
- you eat foods which are not on the list below

If any of these conditions apply, redo the test on another day when you have no extra stress or ailments.

Instruction	Time / Description
Do not take dopaminergic drugs for 7 hours before starting this trial	
1. Wake up in the morning: do not eat or drink but you **can** have a glass of water. Describe symptoms as you awake (e.g. tremor, stiffness, etc). Take one dose of "standard" L-dopa (NOT CONTROLLED RELEASE) and the COMT Inhibitor. Do not eat with L-dopa. Note the time you take L-dopa and COMT inhibitor. Have some dilute apple juice after 10 minutes. Eat Breakfast as soon as the drug takes effect. If you do not have any symptoms as yet, wait until you do before taking L-dopa as per the above instruction. Whilst waiting, eat only fruit (no citrus) and drink herb tea.	Symptoms: L-dopa & COMT Inhibitor time:
2. Write the time of relief of symptoms. Only eat after the drug has taken effect ("kicked in").	"Kick-in" time:
3. Write the time of breakfast (see the specific breakfast menu below) and take the Agonist with a glass of still mineral or purified water. If nausea is a problem, take the Agonist at the end of the meal.	Breakfast time:
4. Write the time of the ***beginning*** of "wear-off " of L-dopa.	Beginning "wear-off " time:
5. Write the time of bowel movement. Describe (difficult / normal).	Time: Difficult/normal

THE SPECIFIC BREAKFAST ON THE EXPERIMENTAL DAY
Eat only the following specific foods at breakfast, immediately after your L-dopa has kicked in. These will not compromise absorption of L-dopa[10,11].

Banana, millet cereal (no other grains added) with water. Cereal can be sweetened with jam or fruit (no citrus). Peppermint or camomile tea. Alternatively, eat vegetable soup (sweet potato, leeks, courgettes, parsley), fruit (no citrus), mint tea.

Resume your usual food and drug regime after completing this trial.
These L-dopa doses on the trial replace your usual first doses of the day.

SCHEME 2(a) **HOW LONG AM I "ON": with L–dopa Madopar 100mg/25mg or Sinemet 25mg/100mg?**

MPORTANT NOTE
Your L-dopa medication will not serve you optimally if:
- you are stressed in any way during the period of this test
- you have a difficult bowel movement
- you are not well (apart from Parkinson's)
- you eat foods which are not on the list below

If any of these conditions apply, redo the test on another day when you have no extra stress or ailments.

Instruction	Time / Description
Do not take dopaminergic drugs for 7 hours before starting this trial	
1. Wake up in the morning: do not eat or drink but you **can** have a glass of water. Describe symptoms as you awake (e.g. tremor, stiffness, etc). Take one dose of standard L-dopa. (NOT CONTROLLED RELEASE). Do not eat with L-dopa. Note the time. If you do not have any symptoms as yet, wait until you do before taking L-dopa as per the above instruction. Whilst waiting, eat only fruit (no citrus) and drink herb tea.	Symptoms: L-dopa time:
2. Write the time of relief of symptoms. Only eat after the drug has taken effect ("kicked in").	"Kick-in" time:
3. Write the time of breakfast (see the specific breakfast menu below).	Breakfast time:
4. Write the time of the ***beginning*** of "wear-off " of L-dopa.	Beginning "wear-off " time:
5. Write the time of bowel movement. Describe (difficult / normal).	Time: Difficult/normal

THE SPECIFIC BREAKFAST ON THE EXPERIMENTAL DAY
Eat only the following specific foods at breakfast, immediately after your L-dopa has kicked in. These will not compromise absorption of L-dopa[10,11].

Banana, millet cereal (no other grains added) with water. Cereal can be sweetened with jam or fruit (no citrus). Peppermint or camomile tea. Alternatively, eat vegetable soup (sweet potato, leeks, courgettes, parsley), fruit (no citrus), mint tea.

Resume your usual food and drug regime after completing this trial.
These L-dopa doses on the trial replace your usual first doses of the day.

SCHEME 2(b) HOW LONG AM I "ON": with L-dopa Madopar 100mg/25mg or Sinemet 25mg/100mg plus COMT Inhibitor?

IMPORTANT NOTE

Your L-dopa medication will not serve you optimally if:

- you are stressed in any way during the period of this test
- you have a difficult bowel movement
- you are not well (apart from Parkinson's)
- you eat foods which are not on the list below

If any of these conditions apply, redo the test on another day when you have no extra stress or ailments.

Instruction	Time / Description
Do not take dopaminergic drugs for 7 hours before starting this trial	
1. Wake up in the morning: do not eat or drink but you **can** have a glass of water. Describe symptoms as you awake (e.g. tremor, stiffness, etc). Take one dose of "standard" L-dopa (NOT CONTROLLED RELEASE) and the COMT Inhibitor. Do not eat with L-dopa. Note the time you take L-dopa and COMT inhibitor. If you do not have any symptoms as yet, wait until you do before taking L-dopa as per the above instruction. Whilst waiting, eat only fruit (no citrus) and drink herb tea.	Symptoms: L-dopa & COMT Inhibitor time:
2. Write the time of relief of symptoms. Only eat after the drug has taken effect ("kicked in").	"Kick-in" time:
3. Write the time of breakfast (see the specific breakfast menu below) and take the Agonist with a glass of still mineral or purified water. If nausea is a problem, take the Agonist at the end of the meal.	Breakfast time:
4. Write the time of the ***beginning*** of "wear-off " of L-dopa.	Beginning "wear-off " time:
5. Write the time of bowel movement. Describe (difficult / normal).	Time: Difficult/normal

THE SPECIFIC BREAKFAST ON THE EXPERIMENTAL DAY

Eat only the following specific foods at breakfast, immediately after your L-dopa has kicked in. These will not compromise absorption of L-dopa[10,11].

Banana, millet cereal (no other grains added) with water. Cereal can be sweetened with jam or fruit (no citrus). Peppermint or camomile tea. Alternatively, eat vegetable soup (sweet potato, leeks, courgettes, parsley), fruit (no citrus), mint tea.

Resume your usual food and drug regime after completing this trial.
These L-dopa doses on the trial replace your usual first doses of the day.

SCHEME 2(c) HOW LONG AM I "ON": with L–dopa Madopar 100mg/25mg or Sinemet 25mg/100mg plus Agonist?

IMPORTANT NOTE
Your L-dopa medication will not serve you optimally if:

■ you are stressed in any way during the period of this test
■ you have a difficult bowel movement
■ you are not well (apart from Parkinson's)
■ you eat foods which are not on the list below

If any of these conditions apply, redo the test on another day when you have no extra stress or ailments.

Instruction	Time / Description
Do not take dopaminergic drugs for 7 hours before starting this trial	
1. Wake up in the morning: do not eat or drink but you **can** have a glass of water. Describe symptoms as you awake (e.g. tremor, stiffness, etc). Take one dose of standard L-dopa (NOT CONTROLLED RELEASE). Do not eat with L-dopa. Note the time. If you do not have any symptoms as yet, wait until you do before taking L-dopa as per the above instruction. Whilst waiting, eat only fruit (no citrus) and drink herb tea.	Symptoms: L-dopa time:
2. Write the time of relief of symptoms. Only eat after the drug has taken effect ("kicked in").	"Kick-in" time:
3. Write the time of breakfast (serve the specific breakfast menu below) and take the Agonist with a glass of still mineral or purified water. If nausea is a problem, take the Agonist at the end of the meal.	Breakfast time:
4. Write the time of the ***beginning*** of "wear-off " of L-dopa.	Beginning "wear-off " time:
5. Write the time of bowel movement. Describe (difficult / normal).	Time: Difficult/normal

THE SPECIFIC BREAKFAST ON THE EXPERIMENTAL DAY
Eat only the following specific foods at breakfast, immediately after your L-dopa has kicked in. These will not compromise absorption of L-dopa[10,11].

Banana, millet cereal (no other grains added) with water. Cereal can be sweetened with jam or fruit (no citrus). Peppermint or camomile tea. Alternatively, eat vegetable soup (sweet potato, leeks, courgettes, parsley), fruit (no citrus), mint tea.

Resume your usual food and drug regime after completing this trial.
These L–dopa doses on the trial replace your usual first doses of the day.

SCHEME 2(d) HOW LONG AM I "ON": with L-dopa Madopar 100mg/25mg or Sinemet 25mg/100mg plus COMT Inhibitor plus Agonist?

IMPORTANT NOTE
Your L-dopa medication will not serve you optimally if:
- you are stressed in any way during the period of this test
- you have a difficult bowel movement
- you are not well (apart from Parkinson's)
- you eat foods which are not on the list below

If any of these conditions apply, redo the test on another day when you have no extra stress or ailments.

Instruction	Time / Description
Do not take dopaminergic drugs for 7 hours before starting this trial	
1. Wake up in the morning: do not eat or drink but you **can** have a glass of water. Describe symptoms as you awake (e.g. tremor, stiffness, etc.). Take one dose of "standard" L-dopa (NOT CONTROLLED RELEASE) and the COMT Inhibitor. Do not eat with L-dopa. Note the time you take L-dopa and COMT inhibitor. If you do not have any symptoms as yet, wait until you do before taking L-dopa as per the above instruction. Whilst waiting, eat only fruit (no citrus) and drink herb tea.	Symptoms: L-dopa & COMT Inhibitor time:
2. Write the time of relief of symptoms. Only eat after the drug has taken effect ("kicked in").	"Kick-in" time:
3. Write the time of breakfast (see the specific breakfast menu below) and take the Agonist with a glass of still mineral or purified water. If nausea is a problem, take the Agonist at the end of the meal.	Breakfast time:
4. Write the time of the ***beginning*** of "wear-off " of L-dopa.	Beginning "wear-off " time:
5. Write the time of bowel movement. Describe (difficult / normal).	Time: Difficult/normal

THE SPECIFIC BREAKFAST ON THE EXPERIMENTAL DAY
Eat only the following specific foods at breakfast, immediately after your L-dopa has kicked in. These will not compromise absorption of L-dopa[10,11].

Banana, millet cereal (no other grains added) with water. Cereal can be sweetened with jam or fruit (no citrus). Peppermint or camomile tea. Alternatively, eat vegetable soup (sweet potato, leeks, courgettes, parsley), fruit (no citrus), mint tea.

Resume your usual food and drug regime after completing this trial.
These L-dopa doses on the trial replace your usual first doses of the day.

SCHEME 3(a) HOW LONG AM I "ON":
with "Stalevo" 50mg/12.5mg/200mg?

IMPORTANT NOTE
Your L-dopa medication will not serve you optimally if:
- you are stressed in any way during the period of this test
- you have a difficult bowel movement
- you are not well (apart from Parkinson's)
- you eat foods which are not on the list below

If any of these conditions apply, redo the test on another day when you have no extra stress or ailments.

Instruction	Time / Description
Do not take dopaminergic drugs for 7 hours before starting this trial	
1. Wake up in the morning: do not eat or drink but you **can** have a glass of water. Describe symptoms as you awake (e.g. tremor, stiffness, etc). Take one dose of Stalevo. RELEASE). Do not eat with Stalevo. Note the time. If you do not have any symptoms as yet, wait until you do before taking Stalevo as per the above instruction. Whilst waiting, eat only fruit (no citrus) and drink herb tea.	Symptoms: Stalevo time:
2. Write the time of relief of symptoms. Only eat after the drug has taken effect ("kicked in").	"Kick-in" time:
3. Write the time of breakfast (serve the specific breakfast menu below).	Breakfast time:
4. Write the time of the *beginning* of "wear-off " of L-dopa.	Beginning "wear-off " time:
5. Write the time of bowel movement. Describe (difficult / normal).	Time: Difficult/normal

THE SPECIFIC BREAKFAST ON THE EXPERIMENTAL DAY
Eat only the following specific foods at breakfast, immediately after your L-dopa has kicked in. These will not compromise absorption of L-dopa[10,11].

Banana, millet cereal (no other grains added) with water. Cereal can be sweetened with jam or fruit (no citrus). Peppermint or camomile tea. Alternatively, eat vegetable soup (sweet potato, leeks, courgettes, parsley), fruit (no citrus), mint tea.

Resume your usual food and drug regime after completing this trial.
These L-dopa doses on the trial replace your usual first doses of the day.

SCHEME 3(b) HOW LONG AM I "ON": with "Stalevo" 50mg/12.5mg/200mg plus Agonist?

IMPORTANT NOTE

Your L-dopa medication will not serve you optimally if:

- you are stressed in any way during the period of this test
- you have a difficult bowel movement
- you are not well (apart from Parkinson's)
- you eat foods which are not on the list below

If any of these conditions apply, redo the test on another day when you have no extra stress or ailments.

Instruction	Time / Description
Do not take dopaminergic drugs for 7 hours before starting this trial	
1. Wake up in the morning: do not eat or drink but you **can** have a glass of water. Describe symptoms as you awake (e.g. tremor, stiffness, etc). Take one dose of Stalevo. Do not eat with Stalevo. Note the time. If you do not have any symptoms as yet, wait until you do before taking Stalevo as per the above instruction. Whilst waiting, eat only fruit (no citrus) and drink herb tea.	Symptoms: Stalevo time:
2. Write the time of relief of symptoms. Only eat after the drug has taken effect ("kicked in").	"Kick-in" time:
3. Write the time of breakfast (see the specific breakfast menu below) and take the Agonist with a glass of still mineral or purified water. If nausea is a problem, take the Agonist at the end of the meal.	Breakfast time:
4. Write the time of the ***beginning*** of "wear-off " of L-dopa.	Beginning "wear-off " time:
5. Write the time of bowel movement. Describe (difficult / normal).	Time: Difficult/normal

THE SPECIFIC BREAKFAST ON THE EXPERIMENTAL DAY

Eat only the following specific foods at breakfast, immediately after your L-dopa has kicked in. These will not compromise absorption of L-dopa[10,11].

Banana, millet cereal (no other grains added) with water. Cereal can be sweetened with jam or fruit (no citrus). Peppermint or camomile tea. Alternatively, eat vegetable soup (sweet potato, leeks, courgettes, parsley), fruit (no citrus), mint tea.

Resume your usual food and drug regime after completing this trial.
These L-dopa doses on the trial replace your usual first doses of the day.

SCHEME 4(a) HOW LONG AM I "ON": with "Stalevo" 100mg/25mg/200mg?

IMPORTANT NOTE
Your L-dopa medication will not serve you optimally if:
- you are stressed in any way during the period of this test
- you have a difficult bowel movement
- you are not well (apart from Parkinson's)
- you eat foods which are not on the list below

If any of these conditions apply, redo the test on another day when you have no extra stress or ailments.

Instruction	Time / Description
Do not take dopaminergic drugs for 7 hours before starting this trial	
1. Wake up in the morning: do not eat or drink but you **can** have a glass of water. Describe symptoms as you awake (e.g. tremor, stiffness, etc). Take one dose of Stalevo. Do not eat with Stalevo. Note the time. Have some dilute apple juice after 10 minutes. Eat Breakfast as soon as the drug takes effect. If you do not have any symptoms as yet, wait until you do before taking Stalevo as per the above instruction. Whilst waiting, eat only fruit (no citrus) and drink herb tea.	Symptoms: Stalevo time:
2. Write the time of relief of symptoms. Only eat after the drug has taken effect ("kicked in").	"Kick-in" time:
3. Write the time of breakfast (serve the specific breakfast menu below).	Breakfast time:
4. Write the time of the ***beginning*** of "wear-off " of L-dopa.	Beginning "wear-off " time:
5. Write the time of bowel movement. Describe (difficult / normal).	Time: Difficult/normal

THE SPECIFIC BREAKFAST ON THE EXPERIMENTAL DAY
Eat only the following specific foods at breakfast, immediately after your L-dopa has kicked in. These will not compromise absorption of L-dopa[10,11].

Banana, millet cereal (no other grains added) with water. Cereal can be sweetened with jam or fruit (no citrus). Peppermint or camomile tea. Alternatively, eat vegetable soup (sweet potato, leeks, courgettes, parsley), fruit (no citrus), mint tea.

Resume your usual food and drug regime after completing this trial.
These L-dopa doses on the trial replace your usual first doses of the day.

SCHEME 4(b) HOW LONG AM I "ON":
with "Stalevo" 100mg/25mg/200mg plus Agonist?

IIMPORTANT NOTE
Your L-dopa medication will not serve you optimally if:

- you are stressed in any way during the period of this test
- you have a difficult bowel movement
- you are not well (apart from Parkinson's)
- you eat foods which are not on the list below

If any of these conditions apply, redo the test on another day when you have no extra stress or ailments.

Instruction	Time / Description
Do not take dopaminergic drugs for 7 hours before starting this trial	
1. Wake up in the morning: do not eat or drink but you **can** have a glass of water. Describe symptoms as you awake (e.g. tremor, stiffness, etc). Take one dose of Stalevo. Do not eat with Stalevo. Note the time. If you do not have any symptoms as yet, wait until you do before taking Stalevo as per the above instruction. Whilst waiting, eat only fruit (no citrus) and drink herb tea.	Symptoms: Stalevo time:
2. Write the time of relief of symptoms. Only eat after the drug has taken effect ("kicked in").	"Kick-in" time:
3. Write the time of breakfast (see the specific breakfast menu below) and take the Agonist with a glass of still mineral or purified water. If nausea is a problem, take the Agonist at the end of the meal.	Breakfast time:
4. Write the time of the **beginning** of "wear-off" of L-dopa.	Beginning "wear-off " time:
5. Write the time of bowel movement. Describe (difficult / normal).	Time: Difficult/normal

THE SPECIFIC BREAKFAST ON THE EXPERIMENTAL DAY
Eat only the following specific foods at breakfast, immediately after your L-dopa has kicked in. These will not compromise absorption of L-dopa[10,11].

Banana, millet cereal (no other grains added) with water. Cereal can be sweetened with jam or fruit (no citrus). Peppermint or camomile tea. Alternatively, eat vegetable soup (sweet potato, leeks, courgettes, parsley), fruit (no citrus), mint tea.

Resume your usual food and drug regime after completing this trial.
These L-dopa doses on the trial replace your usual first doses of the day.

References

1. Professor Aroldo Rossi: 2004: Pharmacological Treatment in Parkinson's Disease: In Dr Geoffrey Leader, Lucille Leader, et al: Parkinson's Disease - The Way Forward!: Denor Press, London, UK: p. 13

2. Bonifati V, Meco G: 1999: New, Selective Catechol-O-Methyltransferase Inhibitors As Therapeutic Agents In Parkinson's Disease. Pharmacol Ther 81 (1): pps. 1-36

3. Rabasseda X: 1999: Prospectives In The Treatment Of Parkinson's Disease: COMT Inhibitors Open Up New Treatment Strategies: Drugs Today 35 (9): pps. 701-717

4. P A Kempster MD MRCP FRACP, M C Wahlqvist MD FRACP: 1994: Dietary factors in the management of Parkinson's Disease: Nutrition Reviews Vol 52, No. 2

5. Lucille Leader: 2004: Optimising Function by Nutritional Manipulation: In Dr Geoffrey Leader, Lucille Leader, et al: Parkinson's Disease - The Way Forward!: Denor Press, London, UK: p. 82

6 Kempster, Wahlqvist: 1994

7. Leader: 2004

8. Kempster, Wahlqvist: 1994

9. Leader: 2004

10. Kempster, Wahlqvist: 1994

11. Leader: 2004

12. Kempster, Wahlqvist: 1994

13. Leader: 2004

14. Kempster, Wahlqvist: 1994

15. Leader: 2004

16. Kempster, Wahlqvist: 1994

17. Leader: 2004

18. Kempster, Wahlqvist: 1994

19. Leader: 2004

20. Kempster, Wahlqvist: 1994

21. Leader: 2004

22. Kempster, Wahlqvist: 1994

23. Leader: 2004

24. Kempster, Wahlqvist: 1994

25. Leader: 2004

26. Kempster, Wahlqvist: 1994

27. Leader: 2004

Chapter 10

Reducing Dyskinesia & Smoothing Out "On-Off" Symptoms

Common reasons for dyskinesia *in some people* can include the following:

1) The *interaction* between *oral* L-dopa *medication* and *protein-rich foods* (for Duodopa, see page 49)

2) The *dosage* of L-dopa medication is too high

3) *Stress* (emotional, other illness, intestinal problems)

4) "*Coming-on*" and "*Wearing-off*" of L-dopa medication

These aspects are presented individually below.

1. The Interaction between L-dopa Medication and Protein-rich Foods
    The clinical experience of the authors demonstrates that some causes of dyskinesia can include the result of the interaction between L-dopa medication and foods which contain the large neutral amino acids. These are constituents of dietary protein. Eating foods which contain these amino acids too close to the time of taking L-dopa, may undermine the effect of L-dopa medication and can sometimes result in dyskinesia. These amino acids compete with L-dopa for absorption through the intestinal wall and again through the blood brain barrier[1].

Continued over page ➡

Commonly Eaten Protein-rich Foods which Compete for Absorption with L-dopa

- Meat, poultry, fish, eggs (*good sources of whole protein*)

- All dairy products including milk, cheese, yoghurt (*but not butter*)

- Soy and pulses

- Wheat (*includes couscous, kamut and bulgar*)

- Rye, oats, barley, spelt, sago

- Coconut

- Nuts, seeds

- Avocado, asparagus

Recommendations

You can avoid this drug-nutrient interaction by following the recommended scheme below:

- Take L-dopa medication

- Eat after L-dopa has taken effect

- If you have eaten any of the dense protein foods in the list above, it is best to wait TWO HOURS if possible before taking L-dopa medication again (only if needed). This is to allow the large neutral amino acids which compete for absorption with L-dopa to clear from their common receptor site in the small bowel.

*If you have eaten other foods, not from the above list, it is suitable to take L-dopa after ONE HOUR

IMPORTANT NOTE

If you are unable to wait for two hours after eating protein before needing L-dopa again, you can replace your concentrated protein food with a *pre-digested* protein drink such as an amino-acid or peptide based drink. Predigested amino acid and peptide based drinks and supplements are more rapidly absorbed than protein in fresh food. These products are therefore helpful when wishing to avoid competition with L-dopa medication within two hours of taking protein. It is usually appropriate to take L-dopa one hour after ingesting amino acids or peptides.

2. Duodopa

    This drug contains L-dopa and is administered by tube directly into the duodenum in the intestinal tract, from where it is directly absorbed into the blood stream. The large amino acids, metabolized from protein, may in some cases adversely affect the efficacy of Duodopa. In these situations, it might be helpful to reduce/avoid food which contains these competitive amino acids during the active hours (see page 48), ensuring the replacement of nutritious alternatives (see page 68-70). However, in order to ensure adequate protein intake during a 24 hour period, protein- rich foods or a pre-digested protein meal should be taken after the pump has been switched off in the evening.

    Note: **Oral "controlled-release" "Slow release[2]"** L-dopa preparations are **not as predictable** as the "standard" formulae, and therefore are not used in this book's drug monitoring schemes. However, they are very useful during the night, in case movement is difficult. To avoid interfering with the absorption of the controlled release L-dopa, subsequent night time snacks should not contain competitive protein (see page 48).

3. The Dose of L-dopa is too High

    If your diet is correct in relation to the times of taking L-dopa, and you are not stressed or constipated - but dyskinesia still remains
    a problem - it is important to ask your neurologist to review the dosage of L-dopa and other dopaminergic drugs since the amount of dopamine being metabolized might be too high.

4. Stress Exacerbates Symptoms

    Many people notice that Parkinson's symptoms are exacerbated by stress. The body needs to produce adrenaline (epinephrine) to cope with stress. Adrenaline is formed (metabolized) in the body from dopamine, which is deficient in Parkinson's Disease! Furthermore, feedback from adrenalin compromises the body's own production of L-dopa. Stress management is therefore important. It is, therefore, prudent to acquire stress management techniques such as those provided by Autogenic Training, Hypnotherapy and Psychotherapy.

5. Smoothing Out "On-Off" Discomfort

Monitoring charts in this book (see pages 30-46) deal with working out how long different doses of L-dopa are effective. The assessment results should be taken to your neurologist who will then be able to advise you of the most effective time intervals at which to take L-dopa in your particular case. The neurologist will also be able to judge which is the smallest dose you can take which will be effective. *Personal experience in our clinic demonstrates that smaller doses of L-dopa taken more frequently can often reduce the "on-off" discomfort and dyskinesia.*

Estimating approximately how often to take L-dopa may be assessed as follows:

IF, for example...

Standard (not controlled/slow release) L-dopa lasts:	4 hours
The time taken to kick-in:	30 minutes
Therefore L-dopa could be taken after an interval of:	3½ hours

References

1. P A Kempster MD MRCP FRACP, M C Wahlqvist MD FRACP: 1994: Dietary factors in the management of Parkinson's Disease: Nutrition Reviews Vol 52, No. 2

2. Professor Aroldo Rossi: 2004: Pharmacological Treatment in Parkinson's Disease: In Dr Geoffrey Leader, Lucille Leader, et al: Parkinson's Disease - The Way Forward!: Denor Press, London, UK: p. 13

Chapter 11

When to take an Agonist, MAO-B Inhibitor, COMT Inhibitor & Stalevo

For drugs which are not listed below, it is recommended to consult the technical advisors of the drug manufacturers concerned in order to obtain information about drug-nutrient interactions and optimal times of taking drugs in relation to food and other drugs.

Agonists – *see Glossary on page 33*

Cabergoline ("Cabaser")
Take Cabergoline as a single dose daily, with food[1]. If patients are nauseous it might be better to take the medication at the end of the meal.

Neupro
As Neupro is an agonist which is worn as a patch, diet is flexible.

Pergolide Mesylate ("Celance")
The manufacturers do not give any guide as to whether this should be taken with or without food. However, it is recommend that agonists be taken after meals if patients tend to be nauseous.

Ropinerole Hydrochloride ("Requip")
Take three times daily with meals[2]. If patients are nauseous it might be better to take the medication at the end of the meal.

The manufacturers state, that as with other centrally active medication, patients should be cautioned against taking Ropinerole with alcohol[3].

Pramipexole ("Mirapexin")
Can be taken with or without food, three times daily[4]. However, to reduce the possibility of nausea, it is best taken at the end of a meal or snack.

The manufacturers state that patients be cautioned against taking this drug with alcohol.

MAO-B Inhibitor – *see Glossary on page 33*
Selegiline Hydrochloride ("Zelepar") / Rasagilene ("Azilect")
Take Selegiline at breakfast as a single dose - or in two divided doses at breakfast and lunch[5]. It can also be taken together with L-dopa. Take Rasigiline as a single dose with L-dopa or alone.

COMT Inhibitor – *see Glossary on page 33*
Entacapone ("Comtess")
Take together with L-dopa ("Sinemet", "Madopar" or equivalent.) If supplementing iron, wait two or three hours before taking Entacapone as it forms chelates with iron in the gastrointestinal tract, impairing drug absorption[6].

'Stalevo'
This drug contains L-dopa as well as a COMT Inhibitor. Clinical experience demonstrates that for optimal effect, take on an empty stomach and only eat after the drug has "kicked in". (See protocols for L-dopa administration presented in this book in Chapter 9.)

As Stalevo contains Entacapone, the same two to three hour interval should be observed when supplementing iron, as it forms chelates with iron in the gastrointestinal tract, impairing drug absorption[7]. Stalevo contains a decarboxylase inhibitor and therefore may be taken with vitamin B6 in the dietary regime.

References

1. ABPI Compendium of Data Sheets and Summaries of Product Characteristics (1999-2000): Datapharm Publications Limited, London, UK: p. 1169

2. Ibid: p. 1609

3. Ibid: p. 1610

4. Website: www.medicines.org.uk

5. ABPI Compendium of Data Sheets and Summaries of Product Characteristics (1999-2000): Datapharm Publications Limited, London, UK: p. 1105

6. Ibid: p. 1104

7. Ibid: p. 1105

Chapter 12

The Compromised Liver

One of the most important functions of the liver is **Detoxification**. During this process the liver detoxifies harmful substances that have entered the body. The liver works extremely hard and performs other vital functions including digestion, building up body tissues, storage of specific vitamins and minerals - iron, copper, B12, vitamins A, D, E and K, whilst also producing immune and red blood cells.

Toxins which are dangerous to the body include those generated from pollution in the environment, insecticides, pesticides (implicated in Parkinson's Disease), alcohol, cigarette smoke, drugs (both medical and street) and car exhaust emissions.

The liver detoxifies harmful substances such as these during two phases of activity known as Phase 1 and Phase 2. In Parkinson's Disease it has been found that Phase 1 may be compromised[1]. It is, therefore, prudent for people with Parkinson's Disease to protect themselves as much as possible from exposure to harmful toxins. Research has demonstrated that individuals who have compromised liver detoxification are more susceptible to developing either Parkinson's Disease or Alzheimer's Disease[2].

It is thought that the rate at which the liver may eliminate toxins can determine an individual's susceptibility[3] to toxic overload, which in turn can lead to symptoms of ill health. The liver can become so overloaded with harmful toxins that the enzymes that break them down can no longer cope. The toxins build up and this may manifest itself as a disease state. Although not everyone exposed to toxins will develop Parkinson's Disease, those unfortunate enough to have an inherited flaw in their detoxification ability are at a far greater risk to the brain damaging effects of a wide variety of toxins[4].

The liver is dependent on specific nutrients for detoxification. These can be provided in the diet. *Specialised nutritional supplementation is available but must only be prescribed by a medical doctor or nutritionist based on each patient's biochemical individuality.*

Detoxification

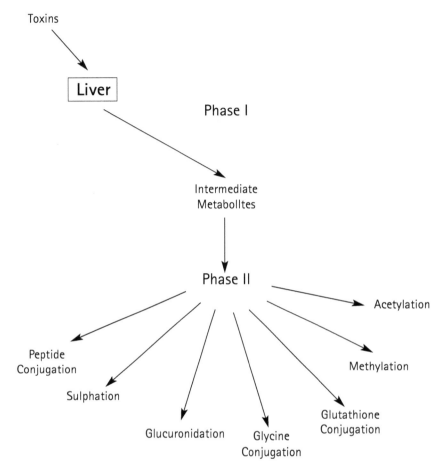

Reprinted from *Liver Detoxification and Optimal Liver Function*: Helen Kimber BSc: *Parkinson's Disease – The Way Forward!* Dr Geoffrey Leader and Lucille Leader (Denor Press)

CAUTION

Popular detoxification "regimes" are not advisable for Parkinson's disease patients. In Parkinson's disease, the liver's ability to detoxify efficiently may be impaired making a detoxification programme completely inappropriate₅. When toxins are released too quickly, this can lead to ill health. However, avoidance of toxins from the diet and eating intelligently, gives many positive health benefits – increased energy, clearer skin, more vitality and a general better feeling of wellbeing. Nutrients which support the detoxification processes (Phase 1 and Phase 2) must only be prescribed by physicians or nutritional therapists.

Dietary Guidelines for Optimizing Detoxification

**An efficient liver detoxification system is vital to health.
This process needs many dietary nutrients.**

- The diet should include plenty of organic, unrefined, unprocessed foods, as fresh as possible.

- Fresh vegetables should include a minimum of one daily serving of the cruciferous vegetables. These are broccoli, cauliflower, brussel sprouts and cabbage. Optimally, five servings of fresh fruit and vegetables should be included in the daily diet.

- Fruit should be eaten but **no grapefruit**, which contains naringenin. Naringenin slows down Phase 1 enzyme activity and a special biochemical test is necessary to ascertain whether people would find it useful or not to include in their diet[6.]

- Nutritious grains include quinoa, millet, buckwheat and tapioca.

- Protein sources can be obtained from fish including herring, chicken, turkey, eggs, nuts, seeds. Red meats should be avoided unless medically indicated and animal fats reduced.

- Do not heat polyunsaturated oils / margarines.

- Sugars and refined foods should be avoided.

- Caffeine, alcohol and other stimulants, could gradually be reduced and can be replaced with delicious fruit and herb drinks.

- Still mineral / purified or filtered water (approximately two litres daily) should be drunk.

- Appropriate nutritional supplements must only be prescribed by physicians or nutritional therapists.

- Corn may sometimes be contaminated by aflatoxin. Peanuts and cashews are affected by mycotoxins.

See over page for **References and Bibliography** ➥

References

1. Williams, Steventon, Sturmann, Waring: 1991: Heredity variation involved with detoxification and neurodegenerative disease: Journal of Inherited Metabolic Disorders: 14: 4

2. Williams et al: 1991

3. Helen Kimber BSc: 2004: Liver Detoxification and Optimal Liver Function: In Dr Geoffrey Leader, Lucille Leader, et al: Parkinson's Disease - The Way Forward!: Denor Press, London, UK: p. 145

4. Williams et al: 1991

5. Williams et al: 1991

6. Great Smokies Diagnostic Lab, Ashville, North Carolina, USA: UK rep Nutri Ltd, Telephone +44 (0)800 212 742

Bibliography

Helen Kimber: Liver Detoxification and Optimal Liver Function: 2006:
Parkinson's Disease - The Way Forward! An Integrated Approach including Drugs, Surgery, Nutrition, Bowel and Muscle Function, Self-Esteem, Sexuality, Stress Control and Carers: Dr Geoffrey Leader and Lucille Leader with Contributions by Prof Aroldo Rossi, Dr Lia Rossi-Prosperi et al. and Foreword by Prof Leslie Findley:
Denor Press, London, UK

Dr David Perlmutter MD: 2000: BrainRecovery.Com: Perlmutter Health Center, Naples, FL, USA

Dr Mark Percival: 1997: Phytonutrients and Detoxification: Clinical Nutrition Insight: Vol 5 No 2

Great Smokies Diagnostic Lab: 1997: Std Detox Profile: Application Guide: Great Smokies Diagnostic Lab, Ashville, N Carolina USA

Mitchell Kaminski MD: 1998: Functional Medicine Symposium - Course Notes: The Gut Liver Connection: Functional Medicine Institute, Gig Harbour, Washington, USA

Chapter 13

Food Intolerance

It is important to identify any food "intolerance" or allergy as it has been observed clinically that eating "problem" food can often exacerbate symptoms. The most common food intolerances noted in clinical practice are:

- Gluten-containing[1,2] grains. These high proportion protein grains are wheat, couscous, bulgar, kamut, rye, oats, barley, spelt. matzo,kamut, durum, einkorn, farina, fu, graham flour, and faro (emmer). The gliadin molecule therein can act as a neurotoxic opioid in some individuals.

- Lectin-containing foods. These are wheat, rye, barley, oats, corn, rice[3], peanuts, kidney beans and other pulses (legumes). They may act as molecular mimics, cause autoimmune reactions[4] and may increase gut permeability in some individuals.

- Casein and lactose - containing foods. These are dairy products. Casein may have an opioid-like effect and the enzyme lactase may be deficient in some individuals.

- Red meat. This can produce inflammatory leukotrines in the gut. Transit time through the intestinal tract is extended due to the specialized demands of protein digestion. The presence of protein over the absorption site for L-dopa in the proximal small bowel, will compromise the absorption of L-dopa[5]. For those who are constipated, the extended transit time is not ideal.

Recommendations

- Clinical observations can be made if a daily diary is used to identify possible reactions to food.

- "Elimination diets" can be helpful: excluding one food at a time for some weeks before reintroducing it again, can allow reactions to be assessed. Always substitute the excluded food with another to maintain weight and energy.

- Tests: There are various types of tests available to identify allergy and intolerance. Doctors and nutritionists will be able to recommend these if the clinical approach is inconclusive.

- Digestive enzyme function should be assessed as incompletely digested food molecules, particularly large protein molecules, may cause reactions. It may be necessary to take digestive enzymes[6] for a limited period.

- Gut permeability should be assessed. Increased permeability of the intestinal mucosa ("leaky gut"[7,8]) may also contribute to immune or autoimmune reactions. This is because the damaged intestinal lining allows incompletely digested larger food molecules to enter the blood stream and they may act as molecular mimics.

    Foods containing lectins have been implicated in causing increased permeability of the gut mucosa by altering tight junction characteristics[9]. This increase may allow passage of normal gut bacteria, pathogens and antigenic partially-degraded dietary proteins into systemic circulation causing persistent peripheral T-cell stimulation.

    If the intestinal mucosa is "leaky," it may be necessary to take a course of nutrients which facilitate repair. These include butyric acid, vitamin C and magnesium. Glutamine in therapeutic doses, usually used for this purpose, may act as an excitotoxin and is contra-indicated in Parkinson's Disease. Vitamin A (which is an aspect of gut mucosal integrity) must only be prescribed professionally. There are serious contraindications for its use in some patients, especially those with a history of cancer, smoking and asbestos exposure. Tests are available to assess the permeability of the gut mucosa.

- Eliminate or rotate offending foods with **substitutes**. However, foods which are implicated in allergy (IgE) should always be avoided.

    Substitutes for gluten grains include: quinoa, corn, buckwheat, tapioca, millet. Corn may occasionally be affected by aflatoxin.

    Substitutes for lectins include: tapioca, buckwheat and millet.

    Substitutes for casein and lactose-containing foods include: nut and seed milks (avoid peanuts and cashews which may contain mycotoxins). If lectins are not a problem nut and seed, and coconut milk/water can be used. Coconut yoghurt and coconut based cheese are also available.

Substitutes for red meat include: fish, eggs and poultry (white meat of chicken or turkey).

It is essential to replace foods which are being eliminated with delicious and nutritious substitutes. Otherwise

there is the risk of loss of energy and weight. Professional nutritional supervision is essential.

References

1. Hadjivassiliou M, Gibson A, Davies-Jones GAB, Lobo AJ, Stephenson TJ, Milford- Ward A: 1996: Does cryptic gluten sensitivity play a part in neurological illness?: Lancet 347: pps. 369-71

2. Auricchio S: 1997: Gluten sensitivity and neurological illness: J Pediatr Gastroenterol Nutr: 25: S7-S8

3. Freed DLJ: 1991: Lectins in food: their importance in health and disease: J Nutr Med: 2: pps. 45-64

4. Pusztai A: 1993: Dietary lectins are metabolic signals for the gut and modulate immune and hormone functions: Eur J Clin Nutr: 47: pps. 691-99

5. Kempster PA, Wahlqvist MC: 1994: Dietary factors in the management of Parkinson's Disease: Nutrition Reviews 52: 2

6. Dr Anthony J Cichoke MD: 1999: The Complete Book of Enzyme Therapy: Avery Publishing Group, Garden City Park, NY, USA: pps. 38-41

7. Ibid: pps. 288-290

8. Kawakami K, Yamamoto Y, Onoue K: 1988: Effect of wheat germ agglutinin on T lymphocyte activation: Microbiol Immunol : 32: pps. 413-22

9. Pusztai A: 1989: Transport of proteins through the membranes of the adult gastrointestinal tract - a potential for drug delivery?: Adv Drug Deliv Rev: 3: pps. 215-28

Bibliography

Pusztai A: 1991: Plant Lectins: Cambridge, Cambridge University Press

Liener IE et al: 1986: The Lectins - Properties, Functions and Applications in Biology and Medicine: Nutritional significance of lectins in the diet: Orlando, Academic Press

Chapter 14

Food Additives
Monosodium Glutamate
& Aspartame

Food to which the sweetener aspartame[1] and flavor enhancer monosodium glutamate (MSG) are added, is best avoided. These products may act as excitotoxins. Research has demonstrated in animals that MSG is implicated in the death of neurones[2]. It is often added to oriental recipes to improve taste and is also found in many other processed foods.

Recommendations

■ Aspartame is used to sweeten food and drinks. Natural Stevia and Xylitol are sweeteners which have a lower glycaemic effect. For non-diabetics, a little honey, molasses, or sugar-free jams are sweeteners. Fruit juice and fruit can also be used as sweeteners.

■ MSG is added to enhance the flavour of the food. Replacing MSG with fresh herbs produces a delicious result and can sometimes stimulate appetite. Restaurants can be requested to prepare food without the addition of MSG.

■ Some people may find that they are sensitive to artificial additives. Food containing artificial colours and non-essential preservatives should ideally be substituted, where possible, with healthier options.

References
1. Russell Blaylock MD: 1997: Excitotoxins - The Taste that Kills: Health Press, Santa Fe, CA, USA: pps. 39-43
2. D W Choi: 1990: Glutamate Neurotoxicity / A three-stage process / Neurotoxicity of Excitatory Amino Acids: FIDA Research Foundation, Symposium Series (Vol. 4): Raven Press, New York, USA

Chapter 15

Free Radicals

Free radicals (reactive oxygen species) form part of protective physiology. However, an excess of free radical production has been implicated in chronic degenerative disease, including Parkinson's Disease. A free radical becomes unstable by having an unpaired electron in its outer shell. It seeks stability by stealing an electron from elsewhere, thus creating another free oxidising molecule. DNA molecules and cell membranes, containing many double bonds, are targeted. Free radical cascade is quenched physiologically by nutrients known as antioxidants. These include vitamins C and E, alpha-lipoic acid, selenium and glutathione.

Excess free radicals are generated by the heating of polyunsaturated fats and oils, surgical trauma, inflammation, radiation[1], disease, drugs[2,3] (medical and social), environmental pollution such as petrol and gas fumes, wood preservatives, fragrance sprays, organophosphates and organochlorine compounds found in pesticides.

How Aspects of Nutrition can Reduce Free Radical Formation

- Potential risks that lifestyle may pose should be reassessed, seeking to reduce exposure to an overload of free radicals.

- Food should be cooked on a low heat, not exceeding 170°C[4.] (Set fan ovens to not higher than 160°C as they reach a higher temperature.)

- Polyunsaturated oils and fats as well as hydrogenated margarines should never be heated. The more stable monounsaturated olive or avocado oil, coconut oil and butter (saturated fat, limited use) are preferable for cooking. Do not exceed 160°C when cooking.

- Food choices should include those which contain antioxidants. These include the bright yellow, orange and dark green fruits and vegetables - sweet potato, butternut squash, plantain, kiwi, dark green cabbage and broccoli are recommended.

Continued over page ➥

- Oral nutritional supplementation of anti-oxidants[5,6] (anti-oxidant therapy) are recommended. These include:

- Vitamins C, E

- Selenium as co-factor for the anti-oxidant enzyme Glutathione Peroxidase

- Zinc and Copper as co-factors for the anti-oxidant enzyme Superoxide Dismutase

- Alpha-Lipoic Acid

- Glutathione[7,8,9,] best administered intravenously or taken orally as its precursor, n-acetyl-cysteine (low doses)

Note: Nutritional supplementation must be supervised by a health professional as some nutrients may be contraindicated in certain pathologies.

References

1. Riley PA: 1994: Free Radicals in Biology - Oxidative Stress and the Effects of Ionizing Radiation: International Journal of Radiation Biology: (65:1): p. 27

2. Werner P, Mytilineou C, Cohen G, Yahr MD: 1994: Impaired oxidation of pyruvate in human embryonic fibroblasts after exposure to L-dopa: European Journal of Pharmacology 263: (1-2): pps.157-62

3. Olanow CW: 1989: Attempts to obtain neuroprotection in Parkinson's Disease: Neurology 49: Supplement 1: S26-S33

4. Udo Erasmus: 1993: Fats That Heal, Fats That Kill (rev. ed): Alive Books, Burnaby, BC, Canada: p. 125

5. Dr David Perlmutter MD: 2000: BrainRecovery.Com: Perlmutter Health Center, Naples, FL, USA: pps. 24-28,30

6. Pong K: 2003: Oxidative stress in neurodegenerative diseases- therapeutic implications for superoxide dismutase mimetics: Expert Opinion on Biological Therapy: (3): pps. 127-39

7. Juurlin BH, Paterson PG: 1998: Review of oxidative stress in brain and spinal cord injury- Suggestions for pharmacological and nutritional management strategies: J Spinal Cord Med: Oct: (21:4): pps. 309-334

8. Oja SS, Jankay R, Varga V, Saransaari P: 2000: Modulation of Glutamate Receptor Functions by Glutathione: Neurochem Int 37: (2-3): pps. 299-306

9. Dr David Perlmutter: 2004: Intravenous Nutrition - Glutathione: In Dr Geoffrey Leader, Lucille Leader, et al: Parkinson's Disease - The Way Forward!: Denor Press, London, UK: pps. 140-143

Chapter 16

Environmental Hazards

a) Organophosphates[1,2,3] have been implicated in neuronal damage.

b) Radiation[4] is implicated in free radical production.

c) Mercury[5,6,7,8] has been implicated in neuronal damage.

Nutritional Therapy Recommendations
Organophosphates

- Avoidance of chemically sprayed foods or other products containing organophosphates and organochlorine compounds. If organic foods are not available, fruit and vegetables should be peeled.

Radiation
- The amount of exposure to the sun and medical X-rays should be monitored. Radiation is also generated during aeroplane flight. Supplementation with antioxidant nutrients may be supportive. Antioxidant nutrients should be supplemented after exposure (with professional guidance), with vitamins C, E, selenium, alpha- lipoic acid. Tests are available which demonstrate cellular levels of antioxidants.

Mercury
- Tests are available which demonstrate levels of mercury and mercury toxicity. If there is medical or dental indication for the replacement of old mercury fillings in teeth, these should be replaced by other materials and chelation therapy[9] administered. There are recommendations for dental personnel who are working with mercury. Research has demonstrated adverse affects on dentists' health due to mercury toxicity[10,11,12,13,14,15]

  However, it is not recommended for all Parkinson's disease patients to automatically have their mercury fillings removed. This process in itself can be detrimental in that detoxification[16,17,18] may be compromised. Advice can be obtained from a dentist practicing specialized mercury removal/dentistry.

See over for References ➥

References

1. Smeh Nikolaus J, MS: 1996: Herbicide 1-methyl-4-phenyl-1,2.3.6-tetrahydropyrinine is implicated in both stiffness and weakness in Parkinson's disease: Save the Children and Yourself – A Guide to a Future Healther Generation by Avoiding Toxins in Today's Food and Water: Alliance Publishing Company, Garrisonville, USA: pps. 189, 266

2. Environmental Protection Agency, Office of Water: 2004: EPA Health Advisory for Hexachlorobenzene: EPA HA d438: Water contaminants (hexachlorobenzene) has been shown to have nervous system effects: pps. 212, 276

3. Environmental Protection Agency, Office of Water: 2004: EPA Health Advisory for simazine (Herbicide): EPA HA d250: Herbicide - nervous system effects including tremor: pps. 225,277

4. Riley PA :1994: Free Radicals in Biology- Oxidative Stress and the Effects of Ionizing Radiation: International Journal of Radiation Biology: (65:1): p. 27

4a. Koutsilieri, E., Scheller, C., Grünblatt, E. et al. J Neurol (2002) 249(Suppl 2): ii01. doi:10.1007/s00415-002-1201-7

5. Perales Y Herrero: 1983: Mercury- Chronic Poisoning: Encyclopaedia of Occ. Health and Safety: 3rd Edition, Vol. 2: Int. Labour Office, Geneva: pps. 1334–1335

6. Ngim CH, Pevathasan: 1989: G Epidemiological Study on Association between Body Burden Mercury Level and Ideopathic Parkinson's Disease: Neuroepidemiology 8: pps. 128-141

7. Rybick RA, Johnson CC, Oman J, Gorell JM: 1993: Parkinson's Disease Mortality and the Industrial use of Heavy Metals in Michigan: Movement Disorder 8: (1): pps. 87-92

8. Ohlson CG, Hogstead C: 1981: Parkinson's Disease and Occupational Exposure to Organic Solvents, Agricultural Chemicals and Mercury - A Case Reference Study: J Scand: Work Environmental Health 7L: p. 252

9. Levenson Dr Jack: 2000: Menace in the Mouth: Brompton Health, London, UK: pps.187-192

10. Shapiro IM, Sumner AJ, Spilz LK, Cornblatt DR, Uzzell B, Shipp II, Block P: 1982: Neurophysiological and Neuropsychological Function in Mercury-Exposed Dentists: Lancet 8282: pps. 1147-1150

11. Ngim CH, Foo SC, Boey KW, Jeyaratnam J: 1992: Chronic Neurobehavioural Effects of Elemental Mercury in Dentists: Brit J. Industrial Medicine 49: pps. 782-790

12. Professor P Stortebecker: 1989: Mercury Poisoning from Dental Amalgam Through a Direct Nose-Brain Transport: (Letter) Lancet 27: p. 1207

13. Cross JP, Daleim Gooluard L, Lenihan JMA, Smith, Hamilton: 1978: Methyl Mercury in the Blood of Dentists: (Letter) Lancet 2: pps. 312,313

14. Ahlbom A, Norell S, Nylnder M, Rodvall Y: 1985: Dentists, Nurses and Brain Tumours 4th International Symposium: Epidemiology Occupational Health, Como, Italy: (Abstracts): Reported Svenska Dagbladet

15. Soderstrom S, Fredriksson A, Dencker L, Ebendal T: 1995: The Effects of Mercury Vapour on Cholinergic Neurons in the Foetal Brain: Studies on the Expression of Nerve Receptors: Brain Res. Dev. Brain Res: 85(1): pps. 96-108

16. Tanner C M: 1991: Abnormal Liver Enzyme-mediated Metabolism in Parkinson's Disease - A Second Look: Neurology 41: (5 suppl 2): pps. 89-92

17. Williams A, Sturman S, Steventon G, Waring R: 1991: Metabolic Biomarkers of Parkinson's Disease : Actor Neurologica Scandinavica : Supplementum 136: pps. 19-23

18. Liver Enzyme Abnormalities in Parkinson's Disease: Geriatrics 46 Suppl 1: August 1991: pps. 60-63

Bibliography

Parkinson's Disease – The Way Forward! An Integrated Approach including Drugs, Surgery, Nutrition, Bowel and Muscle Function, Self-Esteem, Sexuality, Stress Control and Carers: Dr Geoffrey Leader and Lucille Leader with Contributions by Prof Aroldo Rossi, Dr Lia Rossi-Prosperi et al. and Foreword by Prof Leslie Findley:
Denor Press, London, UK: 2006

Chapter 17

Dietary Recommendations for People
Taking L-Dopa

In some foods which contain a high proportion of protein, there are specific molecules (the large neutral amino acids) which compete for absorption with L-dopa from the intestinal tract and also though the blood brain barrier[1.]

Separating the time of any meals that feature these **high protein content** foods from the time of taking L-dopa, may optimize absorption of the drug, rendering it more effective. This will then enable the neurologist to individualise the most appropriate schedule and dosage needed throughout the day.

HIGH PROTEIN Content Food

- meat, poultry, fish
- dairy milk produce (except butter), eggs
- soy, pulses, sago, semolina
- avocado, asparagus, coconut
- nuts and seeds
- Gluten containing products: wheat, rye, oats, barley, spelt, bulgar, couscous, matzo

Less common gluten containing products:

- kamut, durum, einkorn, farina, fu, graham flour, kamut and faro (emmer)

Scheme 1: Taking L-dopa After Eating HIGH Protein Content Food ("Madopar"/"Sinemet"/"Stalevo"/ Zandopa")

Recommendations:

- If you have eaten from the dense protein list above, wait 2 hours before taking
- L-dopa (only if necessary).
- Take L-dopa on an empty stomach (at least 2 hours after eating high protein content food).
- Wait until the drug has "kicked-in" before eating.
- Take a snack or meal immediately after the drug has taken effect. Protein rich foods can now be included as the drug has already entered the brain and therefore there will be no competition at the absorption sites.
- Wait for at least two hours to allow for digestion of high content protein food
- before taking L-dopa again (only if necessary).

Note: If people cannot wait two hours after eating high content protein foods before needing a dose of L-dopa, protein foods *can be substituted* by a pre-digested protein drink - a whey-based polypeptide formula, casein, lactose and gluten-free. Its protein is absorbed more quickly than food and allows L-dopa to be taken after one hour.

Scheme 2: Taking L–dopa after Eating Food which does NOT have a HIGH PROTEIN Content

These foods listed below **do not** appear on the competitive **HIGH PROTEIN Content** List (page 66). They therefore do not pose the same competition for absorption with L-dopa. They contain far less protein relative to carbohydrate.

- fruit
- vegetables (not asparagus, avocado pear, pulses, nuts and seeds)
- fats and oils, butter
- gluten free grains: rice (see page 68 for rice recommendation), tapioca, buckwheat, millet, corn (see page 68 for corn recommendation)

Recommendations:
Having eaten from the list above, wait 1 hour before taking L–dopa (if necessary).

- Wait until the drug has "kicked–in" before eating.
- Take a snack or meal immediately after the drug has taken effect.
- Protein rich foods can now be included as the drug has already entered the brain and therefore there will be no competition at the absorption sites.

Important Observations
In the experience of the authors, these schemes, which take drug-nutrient interactions into account, may be helpful when used in combination with the tools for assessment of dose response (pages 30-46). The neurologist can be assisted in assessing the most affective individualised dosage which may be helpful in the reduction of L-dopa dose-related dyskinesia. Other factors which may induce exacerbated symptoms and which need attention are:

- stress
- bowel function
- other health problems or stressors

Note
If L–dopa takes longer than 30–45 minutes to take effect, consult your neurologist about a form of L-dopa which is more quickly absorbed, for example – a dispersible/liquid form (Madopar Dispersible) or natural brand Zandopa HP200. See over page for Dietary Recommendations ➥

DIETARY RECOMMENDATIONS
"Make food your medicine and medicine your food!" (Hippocrates)
Meals and snacks should be enjoyed! There are always delicious choices!

- ## Eat Three Good Meals a Day and a Snack between Meals
  Meals/snacks may contain protein (taken at specific intervals with L-dopa Medication (see pages 66, 67)), carbohydrates and essential fatty acids.Meals may include sea fish/poultry, eggs, vegetables and fruit.

  Clinical practice finds it helpful to recommend exclusion of:
  gluten grains (wheat, rye, oats unless gluten-free, barley, spelt, couscous, bulgar, kamut), red meat, alcohol, tap water containing heavy metals, the artificial sweetener aspartame, monosodium glutamate, the lectins soy, peanuts and red kidney beans. Delicious and nutritious substitutes are available, **detailed in this chapter.**

- ## Snacks, Energy and Blood Sugar Support
  It is essential to eat a snack containing complex carbohydrate (see page 13) between meals to support blood sugar and energy levels. Protein can be included if the drug-nutrient (L-dopa-protein) timing permits.
  Examples:
  - soup with a base of sweet potatoes, leeks, celery, parsley OR
  - vegetable burgers made with sweet potato, using olive, avocado or coconut oil OR
  - apple puree or just an apple, other fruit, nuts and seeds (high content protein). Nuts and seeds should be powdered if there are swallowing difficulties.
  - gluten free confectionary, toast and spreads.
  - gluten free bread/toast/cracker spread with coconut oil. Coconut oil contains 'medium chain triglycerides' (MCTs) and is a good alternative fuel source to glucose. Glucose as a cell energy source may sometimes be a problem in Parkinson's disease and therefore MCTs may represent an effective alternative energy source to glucose. Coconut oil can also be used for cooking but choose organic type in glass bottles.

Note for Diabetics and People with Cancer
Health professionals must always be consulted for dietary guidance. Rice has a high glycaemic index and contains concerning amounts of environmental arsenic[2]. Basmati white rice contains the lowest level. Arsenic concentrates in the husk of brown rice. Corn contains carcinogenic aflatoxins[3].

Gluten Grains
Wheat, Rye, Barley, Spelt, Sago, Couscous, Bulgar, Kamut
It is noticeable in clinical practice that in some people with PD, grains which contain gluten, are not well tolerated. Some patients notice that their intestinal function may be affected. Their sticky nature, lectin and gliadin portions can sometimes be contraindicated. Gluten sensitivity is common in patients with neurological disease of unknown cause and may have aetiological significance[4].

Substitutes
Quinoa, Gluten free Oats, Corn, Millet, Buckwheat, Tapioca, Teff, Chick Peas (gram flour), amaranth, potato, white rice as grains or in flour form
Rice is gluten free but there are serious contemporary concerns about the environmental arsenic content in the husk of brown rice. Basmati white rice would appear to have the lowest content.

Corn may sometimes be contaminated by aflatoxin, a carcinogen. Soy, although gluten free, is not suitable as it contains lectins, phytates and antitrypsin factors, which may compromise vitamin B12 absorption. The integrity of the intestinal wall is compromised by the ingestion of lectins by increasing its permeability.

Lectins (this only applies to specific medical conditions)
Lectins are molecules contained in grains including wheat, rye, oats, barley, corn, rice, peanuts[5], kidney beans, soy and other legumes/ pulses. These molecules may,

---

Lectins – A Note for Health Professionals
Research has demonstrated that wheat germ agglutinin (WGA) and phyto-hemagglutinin (PHA) from kidney beans increases gut permeability by altering tight junction characteristics[7]. This increase may allow passage of normal gut bacteria, pathogens and antigenic partially-degraded dietary proteins into systemic circulation, causing persistent peripheral T-cell stimulation. It has also been shown that WGA can bind (in vitro) the following tissues and organs: alimentary tract (mouth, stomach, intestines), pancreas, musculo-skeletal system, kidney, skin, nervous and myelin tissues, reproductive organs, and platelets and plasma proteins[8].

Because of their resistance to digestive, proteolytic breakdown, the luminal concentrations of lectins can be quite high. Consequently their transport through the gut wall can exceed that of other dietary antigens by several orders of magnitude[9]. If patients have chronic increased intestinal permeability ("leaky gut"), it could be that foods containing lectins should be avoided until therapy has reconstituted the integrity of the gut mucosa.

---

in some people, cause reactions in neurological and inflammatory diseases as they can act as molecular mimics which trigger auto-immune responses[6]. This is particularly of concern in people with chronic increased intestinal permeability ("leaky gut").

Food that contains lectins can be replaced with other similar types such as millet, buckwheat (kasha), potato and other vegetables.

- ## Vitamins and Minerals
  Eat good helpings daily of dark green, leafy vegetables. They contain minerals which are essential for immune function, bone integrity, cell energy production and which act as important co-enzymes for other cellular functions. Do not cook in aluminium pots. Use stainless steel or glassware to prevent binding of minerals, which reduces their absorption. For valuable antioxidant vitamins which are vital to the quenching of free radicals, include good amounts of red and yellow vegetables and fruit.

  *Greens should include broccoli and dark green leafy vegetables. Spinach, rhubarb, beets and beet tops and Swiss chard not daily due to their oxalate content which can bind to minerals in the gut and prevent some of them, including calcium, from being absorbed, particularly when combined with fibre. Red/ yellow vegetables/fruit include squash, pumpkin, carrot, sweet potato, plantain, mango, papaya, pineapple. Kiwi and apple are beneficial too. Do **not** include grapefruit (see page 55).*

- ## Essential Fatty Acids
  Gamma-linoleic Acid (GLA) and Eicosapentaenoic Acid (EPA) and Docosahexaenoic Acid (DHA). Essential Fatty Acids are obtained from the diet and are used by cell membranes, in immune function and the production of anti-inflammatory prostaglandins.

  GLA is found in mothers' milk, nuts and seeds (exclude peanuts or cashews as they may contain mycotoxins). Keep nuts and seeds refrigerated. Nuts and seeds should be powdered if there are swallowing difficulties. *EPA and DHA are contained in oily fish such as sardines, salmon, mackerel and herring.*

- ## Margarine, Cooking Oil and Fats
  Hydrogenated margarines should never be used. Never heat polyunsaturated oils and fats. Heating transforms them into dangerous trans fats, which can cause free radical cascade. Only in their unrefined, unheated forms can polyunsaturated oils be used, cold, on salads.

Cooking should be with either cold pressed extra virgin olive or avocado oil, organic coconut oil and occasionally butter, if not contraindicated. These oils are the most stable when heated. Keep cooking temperature under 180C with oven and grill temperatures not higher than 160C.

Non-hydrogenated margarines, which do not contain trans fats, may be used as spreads... but must never be heated.

■ Water

Tap water may contain heavy metals and other contaminants.

It is better to drink filtered water or good still mineral water.

■ Red Meat

Red meat can produce inflammatory leukotrines in the gut and takes longer than other foods to be digested and passed through the intestinal tract. It is not ideal food if constipation is a problem.

Substitute with sea fish and poultry, eggs, nuts (do not include peanuts or cashews which may contain mycotoxins) and seeds. Always keep nuts and seeds refrigerated.

■ Animal Milk Products

Except for butter, these are best replaced with other products. This is because casein, found in milk, may be contra-indicated in Parkinson's disease. Lactose intolerance can also cause difficulties.

Vegetable-based milks (almond and coconut) are excellent substitutes. To make almond milk, liquidize almonds and water in a liquidiser. Remember that almonds and coconuts are concentrated proteins. Avoid carageenan in some processed milk as it can be pro-inflammatory.

■ Alcohol

Alcohol can destabilize balance and requires efficient liver detoxification, which can be a problem in Parkinson's Disease. The manufacturers of some dopaminergic and central nervous system drugs advise against the use of alcohol[10]. Gradually and slowly reduce consumption of alcohol by a small amount each week. It is very important not to totally withdraw alcoholic drinks all at once.

Herb and fruit-based drinks can be enjoyed instead and served in wine glasses. Fruit juices should be sugar and artificial sweetener- free and diluted with still mineral or filtered water.

See over for Important Notes and References ➥

■ Caffeine

Caffeine can raise blood pressure and pulse rate and may not be appropriate for everyone. A little in moderation may suit some people. Gradually and slowly reduce consumption, if medically indicated, of caffeine in tea, coffee and chocolate. It is very important not to totally withdraw
caffeine-containing foods and drinks all at once.

Substitutes including herbal teas, green tea and chicory (a coffee substitute) are delicious. Carob tastes similar to chocolate and is a healthy option.

Important Note – Changing the Diet

It is essential that any changes in diet must be made very gradually and carefully. Consult Chapter 19, 'Changing the Diet Gradually and Safely', for recommendations.

References

1. Kempster P A Wahlqvist MD FRACP: Dietary factors in the management of Parkinson's Disease: Nutrition Reviews Vol 52, No. 2: 1994

2. Andrew A. Meharg*†, Enzo Lombi‡, Paul N. Williams†, Kirk G. Scheckel§, Joerg Feldmann , Andrea Raab , Yongguan Zhu and Rafiql Islam. January 15, 2008. Speciation and Localization of Arsenic in White and Brown Rice Grains. Environ. Sci. Technol., 2008, 42 (4), pp 1051–1057

3. Global Burden of Aflatoxin-Induced Hepatocellular Carcinoma: A Risk Assessment: Environ Health Perspect 118:818-824 2010. doi10.1289/ehp.0901388 [Online 19 February 2010]

4. Hadjivassiliou M, Gibson A, Davies-Jones GAB, Lobo AJ, Stephenson TJ, Milford- Ward A: 1996: Does cryptic gluten sensitivity play a part in neurological illness?: Lancet 347: pps. 369-71

5. Wang Q, Yu LG, Campbell BJ, Milton JD, Rhodes JM: 1998: Identification of intact peanut lectin in peripheral venous blood: Lancet 352:(9143): pps. 1831-2

6. Pusztai A: 1993: Dietary lectins are metabolic signals for the gut and modulate immune and hormone functions: Eur J Clin Nutr 47: pps. 691-99

7. Pusztai A: 1989: Transport of proteins through the membranes of the adult gastrointestinal tract - a potential for drug delivery?: Adv Drug Deliv Rev 3: pps. 215-28

8. Freed DLJ: 1991: Lectins in food- their importance in health and disease: J Nutr Med 2: pps. 45-64

9. Wang Q, et al: 1998

10. ABPI Compendium of Data Sheets and Summaries of Product Characteristics (1999 - 2000): Datapharm Publications Limited, London, UK: p. 1610

Notes:

Chapter 18

Dietary Considerations for People
not taking L-Dopa

- It is important to have regular meals and a well balanced diet throughout the day.

- The support of blood sugar levels and energy necessitates a snack between meals (approx at 2-3 hourly intervals).

- Regular bowel function should be facilitated by appropriate fibre and fluid intake.

- It is vital for food intolerances/sensitivities and allergies (IgE) to be identified. The most common food sensitivities noted in clinical practice are:

  - gluten-containing grains[1,2] (wheat, rye, oats, barley, spelt, kamut, couscous, bulgar, sago).

  - dairy produce[2a] (except butter and whey-based casein-free milk drinks).

  - Occasionally all **lectin-containing** foods[3,4,5,5a](wheat, rye, oats, barley, couscous, bulgar, corn, rice, sago, legumes/pulses, peanuts[6]) can be a problem. However, this sensitivity is more likely to occur in those people who have chronic increased gut permeability ("leaky gut" syndrome) and other neurological conditions. **Excluding gluten grains alone, however, seems to be most helpful** in Parkinson's Disease. Medical/nutritional supervision is necessary to advise substitutes for gliadin (gluten) and casein (dairy food[7]).

The general diet, however, should include:

a) **Protein** for the production of neurotransmitters (chemical messengers). Protein is also needed by the body for repair functions. It is found in animal produce, dairy, nuts and seeds.

b) **Carbohydrates** for energy, found in fruit and vegetables.

c) **Essential fatty acids** for the control of inflammation, the immune system, the integrity of cell membranes, memory and other functions. They are found in oily fish, nuts and seeds. Organic coconut oil contains medium chain triglycerides which are used for cell energy. Peanuts and cashews contain carcinogenic mycotoxins so ideally should be replaced with other nuts.

Protein
Fish – sea fish (in preference to farmed fish).
Chicken – (white part, no skin which contains saturated fat).
Turkey – (no skin, which contains saturated fat).

Nuts and Seeds – almonds and other nuts (no cashews or peanuts, which may contain mycotoxins), pumpkin, sesame and sunflower seeds. Keep nuts and seeds refrigerated. *For those who have difficulty with swallowing, nuts and seeds may be hazardous and should be taken in powdered form*

Carbohydrates
Vegetables and fruit are excellent sources of carbohydrate. At least 5 items of fruit and vegetables should be eaten daily. Orange, yellow, red, purple and dark green fruits and vegetables contain valuable anti-oxidants, vitamins and minerals. Do not cook in aluminium pots. Use stainless steel or glassware to prevent binding of minerals, which reduce their absorption.

Vegetables - including sweet potato, carrot, plantain, aubergine (eggplant), courgette (zucchini), green leafy vegetables (broccoli, cabbage, spinach). Spinach, rhubarb, beets and beet tops and Swiss chard not daily due to their oxalate content which can bind to minerals in the gut and prevent some of them, including calcium, from being absorbed, particularly when combined with fibre.

Fruit – including mangoes, bananas, apricots, peaches, melons, grapes, kiwis, pears. However, citrus fruit is contra-indicated if the intestinal permeability is increased ("leaky gut"). Additionally grapefruit, which contains naringenin, should be excluded under particular circumstances (see the chapter on Liver Detoxification – page 55).

Gluten-free Grains
Quinoa, Corn, Millet, Buckwheat, Tapioca, Teff, Gluten free Oats
The above grains are substitutes for wheat, rye, oats, barley, spelt, kamut, couscous, bulgar, sago. Corn may sometimes be contaminated by aflatoxin. Soy, although gluten free, is not suitable as it contains lectins, phytates and antitrypsin factors, which may compromise vitamin B12 absorption. The integrity of the intestinal wall is compromised by the ingestion of lectins by increasing its permeability.

Lectin-free Food (only if indicated by healthcare professional)
Replace lectins with millet, buckwheat (kasha), potato and other vegetables. Lectins[8] are in gluten grains[8], pulses[8], including soy[8], peanuts[8], rice[8], and corn[8].

A Note for Health Professionals
Lectins

There is an interesting connection between foods containing Lectins[9,10,11,12] (grains and legumes/pulses) and increased intestinal permeability ("Leaky Gut").

Grains which contain lectins are: wheat, rye, oats, barley, spelt, kamut, couscous, bulgar, sago, soy and rice.

Substitutes are: **millet, buckwheat** and **tapioca.**

Legumes (pulses) including peanuts also contain lectins.

If the permeability of the gut mucosa is increased ("leaky gut"), some clinicians feel that it is best to avoid gluten as well as lectin-containing grains and legumes. Grains which contain both gluten and lectins are wheat, rye, oats, barley, spelt, kamut, couscous, bulgar and sago. Soy and rice contain lectins but no gluten. It is thought by some clinicians that if the gut mucosa is hyperpermeable or "leaky", the gliadin molecule in gluten could act as a neurotoxic opioid[13], as the principle of the "leaky gut" mucosa may be applicable to the blood-brain-barrier (BBB). Lectins are also best avoided until the gut mucosa is reconstituted, as research has indicated that lectins are capable of disrupting the tight junctions between the cells of the intestinal membrane, causing increased gut permeability ("leaky gut").

Gluten Grains

Research data[14] suggests that gluten sensitivity is common in patients with neurological disease of unknown cause and may have aetiological significance.

Substitutes are gluten-free grains and confectionary. Flours are based on chick peas (gram flour), millet, buckwheat (kasha), tapioca, teff, amaranth, quinoa and potato. Rice is gluten free but there are serious contemporary concerns about the environmental arsenic content in the husk of brown rice. Basmati white rice would appear to have the lowest content.

Essential Fatty Acids

Oily fish (Omega 3) - sardines, mackerel, salmon, herring.

Nuts and seeds (Omega 6) - all but no cashews or peanuts which may contain mycotoxins.
For those who have difficulty with chewing and swallowing, nuts and seeds may be hazardous and should be taken in powdered form.

Dairy Produce

Cows' milk intolerance is often due to a deficiency of the enzyme lactose and sensitivity to casein. The enzyme lactase may be reduced in humans after weaning off mothers' milk, thereby reducing the ability to fully digest dairy food. Casein has been implicated in neurological illness. Dairy is a concentrated protein food which also contains calcium. However, calcium is also found in sesame seeds (halva and tahini) and dark green leafy vegetables.

Dairy substitutes are:

Almond, coconut and gluten free oat milks, and coconut water. Ensure that the products do not contain carageenan, which is pro-inflammatory.

Specially designed pre-digested whey-based polypeptide drinks which do not contain casein or lactose, or pea protein.

Nut and seed milks - made by liquidizing nuts and seeds with the appropriate amount of water. Almonds and coconut can be liquidized with water to make delicious milk. Do not use peanuts or cashews as they may contain mycotoxins.

Butter - after processing, butter is mainly saturated fat and often may not pose the same problem as milk and cheese.

Fluids

Herbal teas, chicory, still mineral/purified or filtered water and fruit juices. Fruit juices should be diluted with still/purified mineral water. Soft drinks, herbal and green teas are preferable to regular caffeinated tea, coffee and chocolate, which contain caffeine and should be taken sparingly if there are medical reasons. There is research which has suggested that coffee may be dopaminergic, but there are other factors which may contraindicate its place in the diet such as hypertension (high blood pressure), tachycardia (fast and irregular heart beat) and stress.

It is vital to drink 8-10 glasses of fluid daily, over the course of the day, to facilitate bowel movement.

Continued over page ➡

Cooking Oils and Fats

Polyunsaturated oils should never be heated. When heated, they become dangerous **trans fats**[15] which can cause free radical damage.

More stable substitutes for cooking are:

Cooking oils, fats - Extra virgin olive or avocado oil (glass container), organic coconut oil (glass container) and limited butter (if there are no other health problems to consider). Do not heat oils higher than 160°C. Temperature will increase in fan ovens.

Spreads – non-hydrogenated margarine (do not heat), butter, vegetable spreads, organic olive and coconut oils.

Food/Salad Dressings – olive or avocado oil and **unrefined, unheated** polyunsaturated oils such as sunflower, sesame and pumpkin seed oils **can be used cold** for food dressings.

Note: Oils, once opened, should be kept refrigerated as they may become rancid. Olive and coconut oils will solidify when cold. They need to be removed from the fridge in time to become liquid and are therefore best stored in a cool spot in the kitchen. Otherwise food can be steamed, sautéed or roasted at low temperatures (below 180°C).

Miscellaneous

Organic food - this is preferable, as exposure to organophosphate sprays is contra-indicated in Parkinson's Disease[16,17]. If not available, non-organic fruit and vegetables should be peeled and washed.

Water – only recognized good-quality water[18] should be drunk. Water purification systems in the kitchen are recommended.

Alcohol – drinking alcohol could present problems as it has been demonstrated that Parkinson's disease patients have compromised detoxification[19,20] processes. It could also be contra-indicated for patients taking other dopaminergic drugs such as Ropinerole[21]. Postural instability (balance) may also be a problem. Consult Chapter 19 (Page 82) for essential **gradual** reduction.

Sluggish Bowel Function

Helpful foods include prunes, figs, cabbage and plenty of fluid. Prunes and figs (dried) should be soaked for a couple of hours until re-hydrated in still mineral or filtered water or gently boiled. If constipation is a problem, two or three prunes or figs are best eaten at 2 or 3 different intervals over the day, between meals, rather than at one sitting (diabetics must be professionally guided). At least 8-10 glasses of still mineral or filtered water should be drunk over the day. See Chapter 8 – Improving Bowel Function (Page 27).

Snacks, Energy and Blood Sugar Support

It is supportive to eat a snack containing complex carbohydrate (see Chapter 5, page 13) and perhaps some protein and medium chain triglycerides between meals to support blood sugar and energy levels.

Examples:

- soup with a base of sweet potatoes, leeks, parsley OR
- vegetable or fish burgers made with sweet potato, using organic extra virgin olive or avocado oil/coconut oil OR
- apple puree or just an apple, other fruit, nuts and seeds (in powder form if chewing and swallowing are not problems).
- gluten free confectionary, toast and spreads (example coconut oil, hummus, olive tapenade).

Special Note: In Parkinson's disease, there can be compromise in glucose and energy metabolism. As such medium chain triglycerides (MCTs) found in coconut oil may be used as an alternative energy source. Oil should be organic in glass containers.

Note for Diabetics and People with Cancer

Health professionals must always be consulted for dietary guidance. Rice has a high glycaemic index and contains concerning amounts of environmental arsenic[22]. Basmati white rice contains the lowest level. Arsenic concentrates in the husk of brown rice. Corn contains carcinogenic aflatoxins[23]. Some oils may be contraindicated.

Important Note – Changing the Diet

It is essential that any changes in diet must be made gradually and carefully. Consult Chapter 19 'Changing the Diet Gradually and Safely' for advice.

References

1. Hadjivassiliou M, Gibson A, Davies-Jones GAB, Lobo AJ, Stephenson TJ, Milford- Ward A: 1996: Does cryptic gluten sensitivity play a part in neurological illness?: Lancet 347: pps. 369-71

2. Auricchio S: 1997: Gluten sensitivity and neurological illness: J Pediatr Gastroenterol Nutrition 25: S7-S8

2a. Millward C, Ferriter M, Calver S, Connell-Jones G: 2004: Gluten and casein-free diets for autistic spectrum disorder: Cochrane Database of Systematic Reviews (2): CD003498

3. Pusztai A: 1993: Dietary lectins are metabolic signals for the gut and modulate immune and hormone functions: Eur J Clin Nutr 47: pps. 691-99

4. Pusztai A: 1989: Transport of proteins through the membranes of the adult gastrointestinal tract - a potential for drug delivery?: Adv Drug Deliv Rev 3: pps. 215-28

5. Freed DLJ: 1991: Lectins in food - their importance in health and disease: J Nutr Med 2: pps. 45-64

5a. Andrew A. Meharg*†, Enzo Lombi‡, Paul N. Williams†, Kirk G. Scheckel§, Joerg Feldmann , Andrea Raab , Yongguan Zhu and Rafiql Islam. January 15, 2008. Speciation and Localization of Arsenic in White and Brown Rice Grains. Environ. Sci. Technol., 2008, 42 (4), pp 1051–1057

6. Wang Q, Yu LG, Campbell BJ, Milton JD, Rhodes JM: 1998: Identification of intact peanut lectin in peripheral venous blood: Lancet: 352:(9143): pps. 1831-2

7. Millward C, Ferriter M, Calver S, Connell-Jones G: 2004: Gluten and casein-free diets for autistic spectrum disorder: Cochrane Database of Systematic Reviews (2): CD003498

8. Pusztai A: 1993, Pusztai A: 1989, Freed DLJ: 1991, Wang Q et al: 1998

9. Pusztai A: 1993

10. Pusztai A: 1989

11. Freed DLJ: 1991

12. Wang Q et al: 1998

13. Millward C et al: 2004

14. Hadjivassiliou M: 1996

14a Andrew A. Meharg*†, Enzo Lombi‡, Paul N. Williams†, Kirk G. Scheckel§, Joerg Feldmann , Andrea Raab , Yongguan Zhu and Rafiql Islam. January 15, 2008. Speciation and Localization of Arsenic in White and Brown Rice Grains. Environ. Sci. Technol., 2008, 42 (4), pp 1051–1057

15. Erasmus U: 1993: Fats That Heal, Fats That Kill (rev. ed): Alive Books, Burnaby, BC, Canada: p. 125

16. Smeh NJ: 1996: Save the Children and Yourself – A guide to a Future Healther Generation by avoiding Toxins in Today's Food and Water: Herbicide (1-methyl-4-phenyl-1,2.3.6-tetrahydropyrinine is implicated in both stiffness and weakness in Parkinson's disease: Alliance Publishing Company, Garrisonville, USA: pps. 189, 266

17. Environmental Protection Agency, Office of Water: 2004: EPA Health Advisory for simazine (Herbicide): EPA HA d250: Herbicide - nervous system effects including tremor: pps. 225, 277

18. Environmental Protection Agency, Office of Water: 2004: EPA Health Advisory for Hexachlorobenzene: EPA HA d438: Water contaminants (hexachlorobenzene) has been shown to have nervous system effects: pps. 212, 276

19. Tanner CM: 1991: Abnormal Liver Enzyme-mediated Metabolism in Parkinson's Disease - A Second Look: Neurology 41: (5 suppl 2): pps. 89-92

20. Williams A, Sturman S, Steventon G, Waring R: 1991: Metabolic Biomarkers of Parkinson's Disease: Acta Neurologica Scandinavica: Supplementum 136: pps. 19-23

21. ABPI Compendium of Datasheets and Summaries of Product Characteristics (1999-2000): Datapharm Publications Limited, London, UK: p. 1610

22. Andrew A. Meharg*†, Enzo Lombi‡, Paul N. Williams†, Kirk G. Scheckel§, Joerg Feldmann , Andrea Raab , Yongguan Zhu and Rafiql Islam. January 15, 2008. Speciation and Localization of Arsenic in White and Brown Rice Grains. Environ. Sci. Technol., 2008, 42 (4), pp 1051–1057

23. Global Burden of Aflatoxin-Induced Hepatocellular Carcinoma: A Risk Assessment: Environ Health Perspect 118:818-824 2010. doi10.1289/ehp.0901388 [Online 19 February 2010]

Chapter 19

Changing the Diet
Gradually and Safely

It can be daunting if your dietician or nutritionist has recommended a change of diet! **The following recommendations are only a guide, should the exclusion or reduction of any food group be advised by a health professional.** They introduce *one* change each week – but of course, the changes can be even slower than that, to suit your own personality and health response. **It is essential to change your diet gradually, under the supervision of a health professional.**

Cautionary Note
Even if you leave out **only one** food from your usual diet, it is absolutely vital that you substitute it with an equivalent. Otherwise, this will result in inappropriate weight loss and lack of energy. It is, therefore, essential to have the supervision of a nutritionist or dietician when you change your diet.

Dietary Change Examples
Many substitute foods can be found at health shops and supermarkets.

Week One: Gluten-free
- Replace

Gluten-containing foods - wheat, couscous, bulgar, kamut, rye, oats, barley and spelt. These are found in pasta, bread, confectionary, processed foods and grain recipes.

- Substitutes

Gluten-free bread, cereals, pasta and confectionary
- products containing potato, white basmati rice[1], tapioca, millet, quinoa, gluten free oats and buckwheat.

Week Two: Lectin-free (medical/nutritional indication only – ref page 76)

- **Replace**

Foods which contain lectins. These are wheat, rye, oats, barley, spelt, rice, corn, soy and lentils. Also kidney beans, other pulses and peanuts.

- **Substitutes**

Quinoa, millet, potato buckwheat and tapioca.

Week Three: Dairy-free

- **Replace**

Milk, yoghurt and cheese.

- **Substitutes**

Animal milk can be replaced by coconut milk and almond milk. Nut milk can be made from liquidizing nuts with water. Keep the milk refrigerated. Soy is contraindicated.

Single cream in small amounts may be tolerated, if cholesterol is not a problem. A small amount of butter may be appropriate but **no** hydrogenated margarine (this contains dangerous trans fats).

Cheese can be replaced by other spreads such as almond or hazelnut butter, olive and home-made vegetable spreads.

Week Four: Alcohol-free

- **Replace**

Alcoholic beverages.

- **Substitutes**

It is **vital** that you **slowly** decrease your daily input by ½ a glass, each week, replacing that amount with diluted fruit juice. It might take up to 4 weeks before you have totally given up alcohol. As you near the end of your reduction period, use smaller glasses for your alcohol and finally, dilute with water.

Delicious non-alcoholic drinks are found in supermarkets, delicatessens or health shops. These are usually based on herbs and fruit. Dilute fruit juice 50% with still mineral water. Serve in wine glasses and chill the juices where appropriate.

Ensure that the drinks do not contain artificial sweeteners. Aspartame is an excitotoxin. *It may need many weeks to gradually become alcohol free.*

Week Five: Red Meat-free

- **Replace**

Red meat such as lamb, beef and pork.

- **Substitutes**

Eggs, fish, turkey or the white of chicken (skin contains saturated fat). Cook with cold pressed olive or avocado oil, kept refrigerated, and only heat up to 160°C. Do not use margarines or polyunsaturated oils to cook with as heating produces dangerous trans fats. You may use a little butter sparingly, if cholesterol is not a problem.

Week Six: Caffeine-free Only if Medically Indicated

- **Replace or Reduce**

Caffeine-containing tea, coffee, cola and chocolate drinks if indicated. For example, people with high blood pressure or anxiety.

- **Substitutes**

NB: Slowly reduce tea, coffee and chocolate drinks by ½ cup only every 3rd day. It is important to replace that fluid with other drinks.

a) Tea replacement can be with Red Bush tea, green tea, peppermint tea or any other herb tea of your choice. Peppermint tea is helpful to the digestion and Red Bush tea tastes like "ordinary" tea.

b) Coffee replacement can be with a pure chicory drink. Make sure that the chicory drink does not contain wheat, rye, oats or barley.

c) Carob is a healthy chocolate substitute.

Research suggests that caffeine may be dopaminergic but there are often contra-indications for taking it due to other health aspects.

Week Seven: Sweeteners

■ **Replace**

Table sugar, refined sugars and all artificial sweeteners.

Typical artificial sweeteners are found in packet juices, cokes and fizzy drinks. Aspartame, saccharine and sorbitol are popular artificial sweeteners.

■ **Substitutes**

Sweeten food with stevia, agave syrup, maple syrup, molasses, dilute fruit juice or sugar free jams.

Week Eight: MSG-free

■ **Replace**

Food-containing MSG (Monosodium Glutamate), which adds flavour. This is an excitotoxin. MSG is often added to oriental and processed foods. It is important to read the labels on food products.

■ **Substitutes**

Herbs and mild spices.

Energy Support

■ **To Maintain Energy**

a) Eat a small snack every two to three hours to support blood sugar levels and have regular meals every 4 to 5 hours.

b) At your mid-meal snack suggestions are, gluten-free bread with coconut oil spread and salad added protein is helpful if this helps the L-dopa-protein schedule. or soup containing sweet potatoes, courgettes, leeks, parsley and tomatoes / apple or apple puree / prunes / figs. A little protein is helpful if this suits your L-dopa protein program.

c) Cook with extra virgin olive, avocado oil or coconut oils. Coconut oil can be used as a spread as it contains medium chain triglycerides (MCTs) which are well absorbed as a cellular energy source. Keep cooking heat low. (160°Celsius) .

A QUICK GUIDE TO ASSIST BOWEL REGULATION
Constipation

- It is better not to eat a heavy meal after 6pm, unless socialising.

- Take a glass of still mineral or filtered water or coconut water several minutes before each meal. Ensure at least 9-10 glasses of fluid spread over the day. Coconut water contains potassium which is helpful to peristalsis.

- At the evening meal, do not eat heavy starches such as (gluten- free) pasta, white potatoes and rice. Rather eat fish, dark green leafy vegetables (limited spinach and rhubarb), and yellow / orange vegetables such as squash, pumpkin, carrots.

- Fruit is helpful, eaten between meals.

- Eat organic prunes or figs that have been soaked (rehydrated) or gently boiled in water. Two or three prunes or figs should be eaten at two to three intervals, spread over the day. Eating these away from meals is best to reduce flatulence. Prunes and figs have a very high fibre content.

- Coconut water, which contains a high amount of potassium, is helpful for intestinal function. Consult a clinical nutritionist or medical professional about the use of magnesium oxide as a stool facilitator and Caricol, which is a papaya concentrate. Supplements which contain senna or cascara are contra-indicated for regular use, as they may cause a condition known as melanosis in the intestinal tract.

Loose Stools

- Consult a medical practitioner in case there are reasons other than dietary for the change in bowel habit. Intestinal disease or parasites may be causative.

- Identify foods which may not be well tolerated and contraindicated as such.

- Apple pectin can slow transit time and bind stools. The medical practitioner must be consulted for recommendations.

Bowel Obstruction

- If there are symptoms of abdominal pain, distension (bloating), nausea and the inability to pass a stool, this may indicate bowel obstruction and must be treated as a medical emergency.

References
Andrew A. Meharg*†, Enzo Lombi‡, Paul N. Williams†, Kirk G. Scheckel§, Joerg Feldmann , Andrea Raab , Yongguan Zhu and Rafiql Islam. January 15, 2008. Speciation and Localization of Arsenic in White and Brown Rice Grains. Environ. Sci. Technol., 2008, 42 (4), pp 1051-1057

Chapter 20

Weight Control

It is important to monitor weight. There could be medical reasons for either weight gain or weight loss.

Considerations for Those Underweight or Those Losing Weight

1. Insufficient daily intake of food.

2. Chewing and swallowing may be a problem, so not enough food is eaten.

3. Difficulty in controlling cutlery, crockery and cooking equipment, so less eaten.

4. Inability to buy, prepare, cook and store food hygienically.

5. Removing offending foods from the usual diet and *not replacing these* with other nutritious substances. This is a very common cause of weight loss in people with Parkinson's Disease who embark upon a new diet without professional supervision.

6. Parasites or infection.

7. Loss of appetite.

8. Malabsorption (difficulty in absorbing nutrients from the intestine).

9. Chronic diarrhoea.

10. "Leaky gut" (increased permeability of the intestinal mucosa).

11. Inadequate digestive enzyme function.

12. Inflammatory bowel diseases (for example – ulcerative colitis, Crohn's disease).

13. Immune diseases (for example – cancer).

14. Other diseases.

Recommendations for Those Underweight or Those Losing Weight

- Consult a Medical Practitioner for assessment/referral to a Nutritional Therapist/Dietician.

- An Occupational Therapist could help find specialized utensils with which to eat and prepare food.

- Foods removed from the diet **must** be replaced with others of equivalent or better nutritional value.

- Tests for parasites or infections if indicated.

- The permeability of the gut mucosa should be assessed (see page 17, Biochemical Tests). If indicated, nutrients for the healing of the gut wall should be supplemented including butyric acid, vitamin C, magnesium. *Glutamine*, although generally prescribed to effect regeneration of the gut mucosa, is *contra-indicated* in Parkinson's disease because, in higher doses, it can function as an excitotoxin. Butyric acid can replace glutamine.

- Food needs to be bought, prepared and stored hygienically. If there is a problem, a medical practitioner should be contacted with a view to referral to a social worker who will find a solution to practical problems.

- It is essential for adults to have minimally 1,500–1,600 calories daily to sustain health. However, it is the quality of the food that is most important. If one is unable to achieve an adequate calorific intake due to inability to chew, nutritious foods can be liquidised. These can also be supplemented with pre-digested complete elemental meals. If swallowing is a problem, naso-gastric or duodenal tube feeding is indicated. This is essential to maintain health and energy.

- It is helpful to have digestive enzymes assessed. This is now possible by non-invasive tests. If there is a deficiency of hydrochloric acid (which digests protein), or reduced pancreatic exocrine function (which digests carbohydrates and fats), supplements of digestive enzymes may be necessary until the condition is corrected.

Considerations for Those Overweight

The following aspects, amongst others, can be considered with overweight.

1. General medical differential diagnosis (different medical causes).

2. Insufficient exercise.

3. Irregular times of eating and excess calories.

4. Food Intolerance / Allergy.

5. Fluid retention.

6. Sluggish metabolism. Thyroid function may be implicated.

7. Hormonal reasons.

Recommendations for Overweight People

■ Consult a Medical Practitioner for assessment/referal to a Nutritional Therapist/Dietician.

■ If exercise is a problem, referral to a physiotherapist or remedial ex- ercise therapist is necessary.

■ The diet should be professionally assessed for appropriate food and calorie content.

■ There may be different medical reasons for fluid retention. Food in- tolerance should also be assessed.

■ Glucose metabolism and lipid profiles should be checked.

■ Thyroid function should be checked.

Chapter 21

Parasites, Co-Infections
and Viruses

Parasites:
Some people suffer from chronic low weight, lack of wellbeing and lack of energy. Neurological symptoms are manifest. Although constipation is more common in PD, there are also those who suffer from chronic or intermittent diarrhoea, pass mucus or blood, flatulence and abdominal distension and experience anal irritation. The causes of symptoms could be as a result of intestinal parasites contracted from food, rivers or drinking water, unhygienic surfaces both at home or whilst abroad.

CoInfections and Viruses:
Other illness could include borellia from tick bites, coinfections from other insects – and viruses including chlamydia pneumoniae, herpes virus types, coxackie virus and others.

Recommendations
The medical practitioner must authorise appropriate investigations.

Tests
Stool samples for parasite detection (at least two to three samples). Blood tests for parasites. These tests are available internationally but Dr Armin Schwarzbach has created a "specialised" laboratory for virus, coinfections and borellia at Arminlab, Augsburg Germany.

Therapy
Drug or herbal therapy, as medically indicated.

Prevention
- Be aware of hygiene in the home. Washing of hands after visiting the toilet or before handling food may be difficult without help and pose a threat to hygiene. Always use liquid soap, individual hand towels and rinse your hands very well.

- Food should be well washed.

- In order to avoid harmful bacterial growth, the temperature of chilled food should be maintained below 34 – 40° Farenheit (below 4.4° Centigrade). Cooked food should be eaten within an hour, after which it should be refrigerated.

- Raw meat, fish, poultry, shellfish and shrimp should be wrapped securely so they do not leak and contaminate other foods.

- It may be prudent to choose only cooked foods in restaurants. Parasites can be found in inadequately washed salads, raw meat, fish.

- Do not eat rare or underdone meat, poultry, eggs and fish. Poultry and eggs, if undercooked, may contain salmonella.

- Always peel fruit when in restaurants.

- Drink purified or recognizable bottled water, especially when travelling.

- Never bathe in "still" rivers or lakes, particularly in countries known to have parasites in these waters.

- Take Probiotics when going on holiday – they may be protective against some bacteria. Probiotics are available from health shops and pharmacies. For travel, choose products which are still viable if not refridgerated.

Chapter 22

Improving Intestinal Environment Generally and After Antibiotics

Antibiotics are necessary for the elimination of bacterial pathogens which cause disease in the body. However, they also destroy the "friendly" bacteria which inhabit the intestinal tract. These friendly bacteria are necessary for immunity in the gut because science has demonstrated that 70-75% of our immune system is to be found in the intestinal tract. This is known as the microbiome. The administration of supplemental probiotics are for the purpose of enhancing the balance of the friendly:unfriendly bacteria which inhabit the gut. Of particular interest in Parkinson's Disease, is the established fact of the gut-brain axis known as the Enteric Nervous System. The health (and management) of the intestinal tract is therefore vital.

Recommendations
A course of Probiotics1 needs to be supplemented if antibiotics have been taken. Cultures of "friendly" intestinal bacteria, which enhance gut immunity, include bifidobacterium bifidum, lactobacillus acidophilus, lactobacillus bulgaricus, saliverius and plantarum. It is best to choose dairy-free products if possible and keep them refrigerated. It is best to check with the technical department of each manufacturer as to whether absorption is best either before or after meals.

A course of Prebiotics may also be professionally prescribed in specific circumstances.

Saccharomyces boulardi should be added to the probiotic administration when antibiotics have been prescribed. It up-regulates secretory IgA and reduces the likelihood of clostridium difficile related diarrhoea

Probiotics
These are Lactobacillus GG/ longum/plantarum/rhamnosus/salivarius/acidophilus, bulgaricus, Bifidobacterium bifidum and other cultures of intestinal bacteria. Each may have its individual indication and contraindication. Gut immunity may be enhanced by these friendly cultures of intestinal bacteria. Prebiotics (nutrition for probiotics), such as fructooligosaccharides and galacto-oligosaccharides, may sometimes be indicated. Brain-derived neurotrophic factor (BDNF) may be enhanced by probiotics, thus positively influencing dopamine metabolism[2,3]

Special Note

Contemporary medical and clinical nutritional thought is that it is best to take a *diverse* range of probiotics and interchange them periodically. There is not yet extensive enough research to indicate the results of long term chronic administration of probiotics and therefore, *intermittent* administration, apart from peri-antibiotic administration, is the preferred option.

Reference

1. Leon Chaitow ND DO, Natasha Trenev: 1990: Probiotics: Thorsons: An Imprint of HarperCollins Publishers, London, UK: pps. 24-25
2. Berton et al: 2006: Nature Reviews Neuroscience 7: pps.137-151
3. Michael Ash, BSc DO ND Dip ION MBANT: 2008: Atypical Depression, The Immune System, Probiotics and Clinical Application: The Stressed Gut - The Stressed Brain: Royal Society of Medicine Presentation: Food and Health Forum: London, UK

Chapter 23

Foods Providing Nutrients

Calories, Quantity and Quality of Food
An adult usually needs approximately 1,600 calories daily in order to sustain health. These calories can be found in quality foods including carbohydrates, fats, proteins, vitamins, minerals and essential fatty acids. Not all foods are suitable for everyone – but there are always choices!

Biotin Egg yolks
Sardines
Legumes (Pulses) – Soy – contains Lectins and may not be suitable, also potentially increasing gut permeability (see chapters 17 & 18 on dietary contraindications)

Calcium
Sesame seeds, tahini – extremely high content
Green leafy vegetables
Molasses
Seafood (be aware of possible toxicity)

Carbohydrates
Grains (buckwheat, tapioca, millet)
Honey
Fruit
Vegetables (sweet potatoes, white potatoes, plantains, squash)

Choline
Egg yolks
Soy - contains Lectins not suitable for increased gut permeability
(see chapters 17 & 18 on diet recommendations)
Fish
Legumes (Pulses) – Soy – contains Lectins and may not be suitable, also potentially increasing gut permeability (see chapters 17 & 18 on dietary contraindications)

Chromium
Honey
Grapes, raisins

Cobalt
Poultry
Green leafy vegetables
Fruit

Copper
Seafood (be aware of possible toxicity)
Nuts (not peanuts or cashews, which may contain mycotoxins)
Legumes (Pulses) – Soy – contains Lectins and may not be suitable, also potentially increasing gut permeability (see chapters 17 & 18 on dietary contraindications)
Molasses, raisins

Cruciferous Vegetables
Broccoli
Cauliflower
Brussels sprouts
Cabbage
Turnip

Essential Fatty Acids (Omega 6)
Nuts (no cashews or peanuts which may contain mycotoxins)
Seeds (sunflower, sesame, pumpkin)
Primrose Oil (only under medical supervision)
Borage Oil

Essential Fatty Acids (Omega 3)
Mackerel
Sardines
Salmon

Mono-unsaturated Fat
Olive or avocado oil ("cold pressed")

Saturated Fat
Butter
Cream
Fatty animal products

Polyunsaturated Oils
Sunflower oil, Sesame oil
(use unrefined or "cold pressed" products, never heat, use for salads)
Margarines (polyunsaturated oils but due to heating, contain contraindicated trans-fats)

Folic Acid
Dark green leafy vegetables
Root vegetables
Salmon

Inositol
Fruit (no citrus if individually contraindicated)
Molasses
Nuts (not peanuts or cashews, which may contain mycotoxins)
Vegetables

Iron
Egg Fish Poultry
Blackstrap molasses
Cherry juice
Green leafy vegetables
Dried fruits

Magnesium
Seafood (be aware of possible toxicity)
Dark green vegetables
Molasses
Nuts (not peanuts or cashews, which may contain mycotoxins)

Manganese
Green leafy vegetables
Legumes (Pulses) – Soy – contains Lectins and may not be suitable, also potentially increasing gut permeability (see chapters 17 & 18 on dietary contraindications)
Nuts (not peanuts or cashews, which may contain mycotoxins)
Pineapples
Egg yolks

Molybdenum
Legumes (Pulses) – Soy – contains Lectins and may not be suitable, also potentially increasing gut permeability (see chapters 17 & 18 on dietary contraindications)
Dark green vegetables

Para-Aminobenzoic Acid (PABA)
Molasses
Green leafy vegetables

Phosphatidyl Choline (lecithin)
Sunflower lecithin
Eggs (yolks)

Phosphorous
Fish
Poultry
Egg
Legumes (Pulses) – Soy – contains Lectins and may not be suitable, also potentially increasing gut permeability (see chapters 17 & 18 on dietary contraindications)
Nuts (not peanuts or cashews, which may contain mycotoxins)

Polyphenols
Red grapes (with skin)

Potassium
Legumes (Pulses) – Soy – contains Lectins and may not be suitable, also potentially increasing gut permeability (see chapters 17 & 18 on dietary contraindications)
Sunflower seeds

Protein
Fish, Poultry, Egg
Soy – contains Lectins and may not be suitable, also potentially increasing gut permeability (see chapters 17 & 18 on dietary contraindications)

Selenium
Herring
Sesame seeds

Sodium
Seafood (be aware of possible toxicity)

Sulphur
Fish, Garlic, Onions, Egg, Cabbage
Horseradish

Tryptophane
Bananas

Vanadium
Fish

Vitamin A (beta-carotene sources yielding vitamin A)
Red and yellow fruits (apricot, mango, papaya, cherry, peach, watermelon)
Dark green vegetables (kale, romaine lettuce, beet greens, parsley)
Yellow vegetables (carrots, sweet potatoes, pumpkin, tomatoes)
Red cabbage, Eggs

Vitamin B1
Blackstrap molasses
Fish
Poultry
Egg yolks
Legumes (Pulses) – Soy – contains Lectins and may not be suitable, also potentially increasing gut permeability (see chapters 17 & 18 on dietary contraindications)
Nuts (not peanuts or cashews, which may contain mycotoxins)

Vitamin B2
Blackstrap molasses
Egg yolks
Legumes (Pulses) – Soy – contains Lectins and may not be suitable, also potentially increasing gut permeability (see chapters 17 & 18 on dietary contraindications)
Nuts (not peanuts or cashews, which may contain mycotoxins)

Vitamin B3 (Niacin)
Poultry
Fish

Vitamin B5 (Pantothenic Acid)
Egg yolks
Legumes (Pulses) – Soy – contains Lectins and may not be suitable, also potentially increasing gut permeability (see chapters 17 & 18 on dietary contraindications)
Salmon

Vitamin B6
Blackstrap molasses
Legumes (Pulses) – Soy – contains Lectins and may not be suitable, also potentially increasing gut permeability (see chapters 17 & 18 on dietary recommendations)
Green leafy vegetables

Vitamin B12 (vitamin B12 supplementation possibly necessary for vegetarians)
Fish
Egg
Unprocessed spirulina

Vitamin C
Fruit (no citrus if individually contraindicated)
Rose hips, tomatoes
Acerola cherries
Cantaloupe melon
Strawberries
Kiwi
Broccoli
Green peppers

Vitamin D
Salmon
Sardines
Herring
Egg yolks

Vitamin E
Cold pressed oils
Egg
Molasses
Sweet potatoes

Vitamin K
Cauliflower
Green leafy vegetables
Egg
Safflower oil
Blackstrap molasses
Soy – contains Lectins and may not be suitable, also potentially increasing gut permeability (see chapters 17 & 18 on dietary recommendations)
Fruit (no citrus if individually contraindicated)
Blackcurrants
Buckwheat
Mushrooms
Herring

Water
Mineral water
Purified water

Zinc
Pumpkin seeds
Sunflower seeds
Sesame seeds
Seafood (be aware of possible toxicity)

Bibliography

Gayla J Kirschmann, John D Kirschmann: 1996: Nutrition Almanac 4th edition: McGraw-Hill, New York, USA

McCance and Widdowson's: 1993: The Royal Society of Chemistry & Ministry of Agriculture, Fisheries and Food: The Composition of Foods: Zerox Ventura, Cambridge, UK

Chapter 24

A Natural Source of L-Dopa

"Zandopa"(HP 200)

L-dopa derived from a plant source (mucuna pruriens) has been found in clinical trials[1,2,3,4,5,6] to be effective in the control of symptoms of Parkinson's Disease. Some patients are prescribed this form of medication by their neurologists if they are unable to tolerate pharmaceutical L-dopa and in some cases it may be helpful. Doses of L-dopa from mucuna pruriens have been standardized in a specialised manufacturing process. As with other drugs and nutrients, consideration must be given to possible drug - nutrient interactions or contraindications for its use due to specific health conditions. Long-term effects must still be medically evaluated. As such, **administration and monitoring of mucuna pruriens must always be under medical supervision. It should only be bought from a recognized pharmaceutical source with high-grade manufacturing standards. It is best taken following the general dietary recommendations for L-dopa pharmaceutical medication.** The product Zandopa: HP200 contains standardised L-dopa from mucuna pruriens.

Important Note

Patients must not "self medicate" or use the unprocessed mucuna pruriens beans as a vegetable, as there can be associated health risk.

References

1. Manyam BV, et al: 1995: The Journal of Alternative and Complementary Medicine: Volume 1, nr 3: An Alternative Medicine Treatment for Parkinson's Disease: Results of a Multicenter Clinical Trial - HP-200 in Parkinson's Disease Study Group: pps. 249-255

2. Manyam BV, Sanchez-Ramos JR: 1999: Traditional and Complementary Therapies in Parkinson's Disease: Adv Neurol. 80: pps. 565-74

3. Nagashayana N, Sankarankutty P, Nampoothiri MR, Mohan PK, Mohanakumar KP: 2000: Association of L-DOPA with Recovery following Ayurveda Medication in Parkinson's disease: J Neurol Sci. 15: 176(2): pps. 124-7

4. Singhal B, Lalkaka J, Sankhla C: 2003: Epidemiology and Treatment of Parkinson's disease in India: Parkinsonism Relat Disord: Suppl 2: S105-9

5. Manyam BV, Dhanasekaran M, Hare TA: 2004: Effect of Antiparkinson Drug HP-200 (Mucuna pruriens) on the central monoaminergic neurotransmitters: Phytother Res: 18(2): pps. 97-101

6. *J Neurol Neurosurg Psychiatry* 2004;75:1672-1677 doi:10.1136/jnnp.2003.028761 *Mucuna pruriens* in Parkinson's disease: a double blind clinical and pharmacological study R Katzenschlager[1,2], A Evans[1], A Manson[3], P N Patsalos[4], N Ratnaraj[4], H Watt[5],L Timmermann[6], R Van der Giessen[7], A J Lees[1]

Chapter 25

Safety and Hygiene in the Kitchen

Basic Hygiene
Hands must be thoroughly soaped and rinsed under running water before preparing food. It is best to use liquid soap and disposable towels. Hair and loose clothing should be restrained to avoid contamination.

Why Worry About Temperature?
All food is subject to bacteria. To avoid growth of harmful bacteria (between 21-49°C/70-120°F), food should be kept either refrigerated or properly hot after cooking, and not left at room temperature for any length of time.

Food Preparation
It is best to defrost frozen foods slowly in the refrigerator. Otherwise this can be done under cold, running, drinking water or in a microwave oven. Do not delay between defrosting and cooking.

Always ensure food preparation tools (knives, cutting boards, pans etc.) are washed and well rinsed. When preparing food, keep raw foods away from cooked foods. Rinse all food properly before use.

It is practical to prepare individual portions of food which can be cooked/reheated as needed. If refrigerating cooked food, chill to below 8°C/46°F before sealing.

Ensure food is thoroughly cooked, especially meat, poultry, fish and eggs. Food and cooking oils should not be heated/cooked beyond 160oC (fan ovens usually heat up to a higher temperature) to avoid the production of transfats and other harmful substances.

Food Storage and Reheating and Serving
Food should be kept in a well-regulated refrigerator or freezer until needed for cooking or eating. Do not eat food with mould or which is older than its "use-by" date. Refrigerated, cooked food should be eaten within two days.

Food must be reheated throughout and served piping hot. Heat to at least 74°C/165°F. Take extra care when reheating cooked food that has been chilled. Maintain hot cooked food at 63°C/145°F until eaten.

Emergency Supplies

Always have some tinned and frozen food available for emergencies. For example: mackerel, sardines, green and orange vegetables, fruit and soups. Tuna and swordfish contain a high amount of environmental mercury so are not recommended. Corn, peanuts and cashews contain aflatoxins and therefore alternatives are more suitable,

If Cooking is Difficult, Occupational Therapist

If food preparation is difficult, specialist organizations, supermarkets and shops can help with provision and delivery of meals.

If movement is hazardous, a microwave oven may be the only solution. However, for optimal health, it would certainly be better to use conventional methods of cooking. An electric tin opener may be helpful as well as an electric mixer and blender.

Occupational Therapists can identify physical challenges in the home and provide solutions. They can recommend helpful aids, such as specialized eating utensils, as well as chairs, beds and baths.

Social Worker, Help and Hygiene

It is essential to maintain kitchen cleanliness. An automatic dishwasher may be helpful. Referral to a Social Worker can help in finding a support team to assist with any special needs.

Fire

Safety requires a fire blanket or fire extinguisher to be easily accessible and able to be used in an emergency. A smoke alarm is essential both in the kitchen and in other areas in the home.

Emergency Call

In case of emergency it is helpful to wear and operate a 'panic button' linked to a central call station. This can be organized by an occupational therapist or social worker.

Bibliography

http://www.opsi.gov.uk/si/si1995/Uksi_19952200_en_1.htm#end The Food Standards Agency: http://www.food.gov.uk/
http://www.metrokc.gov/HEALTH/foodsfty/kitchensafety.htm

Chapter 26

Recipes for all Occasions!

These delicious and simple recipes are suitable for use whether L-dopa medication is used or not. They are gluten and dairy free.

The recipes are also suitable for family and friends!

Bon Appetit!

SOUPS

Satisfying Sweet Potato Soup
3 sweet potatoes 1 large onion / leek
1 zucchini (courgette) 1 bunch parsley
1 litre of water 2 tomatoes
Small amount of Kale and broccoli

1. Boil all the ingredients in 1 litre of purified or still mineral water.
   Cover and simmer on low heat.

2. As soon as vegetables are soft, remove from the water. Liquidize or blend in a food processor. Add the vegetable water to make up the desired consistency of the soup.

Gazpacho Soup
5 large tomatoes   1 clove garlic
½ cup green pepper   1 cup cucumber
1 cup tomato juice   ½ cup sweet red pepper
2 tbsp olive or avocado oil (cold-pressed)   ½ cup fresh parsley
Black pepper (optional)   2 tsp basil

1. Combine all ingredients and liquidize or blend in a food processor.
   Serve chilled.

SALADS

Potato Salad
4 potatoes (in skins, if organic)
2 spring onions (chopped)
sprinkling of chives (chopped)
garlic and black pepper
dressing made with 3 tbsp cold pressed olive or avocado oil
and 1 tbsp lemon juice (or tomato juice)

1. Mix the ingredients together in a bowl and toss with the Mediterranean Dressing. Mayonnaise can also be used as a dressing during a "protein window" and/or chopped or grated hardboiled egg.

Fresh Mixed Salad
pepper (red, green or yellow)
tomatoes (finely sliced) lettuce
finely grated carrot cucumber

1. Dressing made with 3 tbsp cold pressed olive or avocado oil and 1 tbsp lemon juice (or tomato juice), crushed garlic and black pepper to taste.

Carrot Salad
Grate carrots finely and dress with soaked sultanas and pineapple juice, or serve plain.

SALAD DRESSING

Mediterranean Dressing
6 tbsp cold pressed olive or avocado oil
(remove from the fridge 10 minutes before use)
3 tbsp lemon juice or tomato juice
1 pressed garlic clove or garlic grains (to taste - optional)
ground black pepper

1. Mix all the ingredients together and stir – or shake if in a closed bottle.

GRAIN RECIPES
(GLUTEN FREE)

White Basmati Rice

1 cup white rice (research[1] demonstrates that brown rice tends to have higher levels of environmental arsenic which may not be optimal for human health.)
2½ cups water (purified or still mineral water)

1. Wash rice 3 times in cold water
2. Put rice and water together in a pot
3. Bring to boil
4. Stir once
5. Put lid on and simmer on a low heat for 20 minutes

Countryside Peppers

6 medium red/yellow/orange peppers
3 cups water (purified or still mineral water)
1 cup millet
1 ½ cups onion, chopped
1 clove garlic, crushed
½ cup mushrooms, diced
1 tbsp olive or avocado oil (cold-pressed)
crushed black pepper (optional)

1. Blanch peppers in boiling water. Allow to cool slightly.

2. Bring water and millet to a boil. Reduce heat. Cover and simmer

3. In a pan, heat oil and sauté garlic, onion and mushrooms. Season to taste.

4. Combine cooked millet, and add to onion mixture.

5. Fill peppers with millet mixture. Cover with a little cold pressed olive or avocado oil.

6. Bake at 160°C for approximately 40 minutes or until the peppers are soft.

BREADS

Sweet Potato and Oregano Bread (makes 1 x 1lb loaf)
(Harriet Jedwab)

Dough:

175g (6oz) peeled, cored coarsely grated sweet potato) have this ready before you start
1½ tbsp of extra virgin olive oil
2 heaped tsps dried oregano (or 3 heaped tbsp chopped fresh oregano)
1 heaped tsp dried thyme or 2 tbsp chopped fresh thyme
225g (8 oz) Doves Farm gluten-free flour
3 level tsp gluten-free baking powder
2 large egg egg yolks, lightly beaten with 2-3 tbsp almond milk (must not contain carageenan). If dough still feels dry, add a little extra almond milk.

1. Preheat oven to 160°C

2. Lightly grease a 1lb loaf tin (glass) and line with a piece of greaseproof paper, long enough to hang over the two long sides, by 50-70mm (2-3") - as a 'scoop', to lift the baked bread out of the tin.

3. Sift flour, baking powder, dried herbs into a large bowl.

4. Add grated sweet potato and mix together, with a wooden/metal spoon.

5. Add olive oil plus egg and milk mixture, a little at a time, until a loose, sticky dough is formed - if necessary add a couple more tablespoons of milk to the mixture and finish mixing with your hands, to form a "loaf" shape to go into the loaf tin or a round blob to sit on the baking tray.

6. Transfer to the the lined loaf tin/baking tray and bake in the oven, for 45-50 minutes, until golden and crusty.

7. Remove from tin and cool on a wire rack (or serve warm).

Nut Bread

1 tea cup almond flour
1 tea cup walnuts, chopped
3 eggs or 2 level tablespoons tapioca flour if eggs are contraindicated
A little coconut water or almond milk may be necessary to reach a soft consistency
2½ flat tablespoons Coconut oil (melt)
2 bananas, not over-ripe

1. In food processor, put the eggs and bananas. When blended (roughly) remove to a mixing bowl and add the dry ingredients. Add in the melted coconut oil. Mix all together well and pour into an oven dish, well oiled with coconut oil.

2. Heat oven to 155°C and bake for 40/45 minutes. Allow to cool completely before removing from dish as it is rather crumbly.

GRAIN RECIPES
(LECTIN & GLUTEN-FREE)

Savoury Pancakes/Crepes *with* Eggs (high protein)
(Marta Bucko)

To be used as sweet or savory wraps, for all occasions
40 grams buckwheat flour
60 grams millet flour (or flakes)
2 eggs
1 tbs water
olive or avocado oil or butter

1. Beat eggs.
2. Gradually add to flour, stirring all the time.
3. Add water, whilst still stirring.
4. Heat the pan, greased with olive or avocado oil or butter.
5. Add the mixture to cover the bottom of the pan.
6. Lower the heat.
7. Turn the pancake over when bubbles are seen on its surface.
8. Cook to a golden-brown color.
9. Serve with jam, honey, ratatouille or any other spread preferred.

Continued over page ➥

Sweet Pancakes/Crepes *without* Eggs (negligible protein content)
(Marta Bucko)

To be used as sweet or savory wraps for all occasions.

40 grams buckwheat flour
60 grams millet flour (or flakes)
1 heaped tbs jam
1 tbs water
olive or avocado oil or butter

1. Put flour in large mixing bowl.
2. Fold jam into the flour.
3. Add water, whilst still stirring.
4. Heat the pan, greased with olive or avocado oil or butter.
5. Add the mixture to cover the bottom of the pan.
6. Lower the heat.
7. Turn the pancake over when bubbles are seen on its surface.
8. Cook to a golden-brown color.
9. Serve with jam, honey, mashed banana, other fruit or vegetable spread.

Millet or Quinoa or Gluten free Oats Porridge
4 tbs millet flakes
water to cover the flakes
add organic maple syrup and/or fresh fruit – to taste, after cooking

1. Put the flakes into a small pot on the stove.

2. Slowly add the water, whilst stirring, to prevent any lumps being formed.

3. Bring the mixture to the boil, whilst still stirring, and then immediately lower the heat.

4. Keep stirring for a minute or two until the porridge has reached the desired consistency.

5. Serve with spoonfuls of jam/honey or sliced fruit – to taste.

6. Eat millet intermittently, not on a daily basis.

PASTA
(GLUTEN-FREE)

Salmon Surprise a la Ray
(Rachael Leader: Fail-Safe Recipes)

half packet of basmati white rice (see page 68 for details on rice)
or buckwheat noodles (gluten-free noodles)
2 small tins of wild salmon in spring water or olive or avocado oil
1 tbsp. cold pressed olive or avocado oil (if not using wild salmon with olive
or avocado oil)
juice of half a lemon

1. Cover noodles generously with water.

2. Boil gently with the lid off, stirring regularly.

3. Flake the tuna and mix into the cooked noodles.

4. The Dressing: mix a little cold pressed olive or avocado oil and lemon through the noodles or use 1tbs. organic mayonnaise and 2tbs. Heinz Tomato Ketchup (mixed to taste)

5. Alternatively: vegetables can be stir-fried in olive or avocado oil and mixed into the noodles – without wild salmon. This combination will therefore not contain a competitive protein level with L-dopa.

Continued over page ➻

POTATOES
(SWEET AND PLAIN)

Potato Cakes
4 medium potatoes (2 sweet and 2 plain)
1 egg
2 onions
1 tbsp. buckwheat flour
2 tbsp quinoa
2 tbsp. olive or avocado oil (cold-pressed)

1. First chop the potatoes and onions into quarters. Place in a food processor together with the flour/quinoa, egg and 2 tbsp. of olive or avocado oil. Chop to a fine, coarse mixture (do not allow to become liquid). If watery, add a little more flour, so that the consistency does not fall apart, but is still soft.

2. Heat a frying pan or griddle with a dash of olive or avocado oil, sufficient so that the cakes will not stick to the bottom. Keep heat at medium setting.

3. Drop the mixture by the dessertspoon onto a pan or onto griddle, cover but keep checking to make sure cakes don't burn or stick.

   Flip over when lightly browned and cook underside. Total cooking time may vary. These are like little potato burgers.

Alternative Method

4. The cakes may be baked. Lightly grease an oven dish or baking tin with cold pressed olive or avocado oil. Drop spoonfuls of potato mixture into the dish and pour a little olive or avocado oil over each one. Cover with tin foil, not touching the food. Bake at 160°C until the potato is cooked through. Remove the tin foil about 5 minutes before serving, in order to crisp.

Jacket Potatoes

organically grown potatoes, sweet or plain
olive or avocado oil
butter

1. Scrub clean the skins of sweet or ordinary potatoes and prick the potatoes with a fork. (If not organic, potatoes must be peeled).

2. Brush potatoes with a little olive or avocado oil and wrap first in greaseproof paper and then in aluminum foil. Caution: Make sure that the aluminum foil completely covers the greaseproof paper or it will catch alight in the oven!

3. Bake in the oven at 160°C for an hour and a half, or until soft.

4. Serve with butter, salad or vegetables.

Roast Potatoes

6 sweet or plain potatoes with skin on (if not organic, potatoes must be peeled).
(pumpkin or butternut squash can also be used)
olive or avocado oil rosemary

1. Steam potatoes until soft and place in an open oven dish. Use the water left over later in soup.

2. Coat potatoes with cold-pressed olive or avocado oil. Sprinkle fresh or dried rosemary over the potatoes.

3. Roast in the oven at 160°C for approximately 1½ hours.

Tomato Sauce

2 tbs olive or avocado oil (cold-pressed)
1 clove garlic, crushed
1 medium onion/leek, chopped 1 lb. chopped tomatoes
3 tbs. tomato puree

1. Bring the water to a boil in a large saucepan. Gradually add it to the cornmeal, continually stirring to avoid lumps. Add butter, continuing to cook over a low flame for 20 minutes. The mixture should have a creamy consistency. If not, it may be necessary to add more butter/water.

2. Pour into a 13 x 9 inch baking tin, level and set aside to cool.

3. Prepare sauce by heating oil in a saucepan, sauté garlic and onion till tender, then add oregano, basil, fennel seeds and black pepper. Stir in chopped tomatoes and puree, add fructose, cover and simmer for 20-30 minutes or until sauce thickens.

FISH and POULTRY

Tomato Chicken

4 breasts of chicken / turkey or whole chicken
200ml or 1 large english tea cup Heinz Tomato Sauce
1 cup purified or still mineral water
4 - 6 dessertspoonful cold pressed olive or avocado oil
2 onions or 1 leek, chopped herbs of choice
4 plain & 4 sweet potatoes, whole/sliced
2 apples, quartered (optional)

1. Mix tomato sauce, oil and water together. Pour this mixture over the chicken and vegetables. If you do not have enough gravy to cover chicken and potatoes, add a little more tomato sauce and water.

2. Bake in oven at 160°C, in a tightly covered dish, for about 2 hours or until the chicken is soft.

3. Note: This dish can also be cooked on top of the stove, in a covered pot, at a low temperature, for approximately 1½ hours or until the chicken and vegetables are tender. Check sauce level frequently, adding a little water if necessary to maintain sufficient liquid. Stir intermittently.

Mediterranean Fish

1 fillet of plaice / cod or other fish black pepper
pressed fresh garlic or garlic granules cold pressed olive or avocado oil
½ lemon

1. Lace the frying pan with cold pressed olive or avocado oil and the juice of ½ of the lemon.

2. Put the remaining shell of the lemon, (open side down) in the olive or avocado oil and lemon mixture.

3. Using low heat, when beginning to cook, place fish in the pan.

4. Put the lid on the pan and allow to cook through on a low heat.

5. Check continuously that the mixture is not drying out and turn the fish, if necessary.

6. Cook for 15 minutes or until the fish is properly cooked through.

Note: This dish could also be baked in an oven in a tightly covered dish for 1 hour at 160°C.

Continued over page ➡◆

DESSERTS
(DAIRY AND GLUTEN FREE)

Exotic Coconut Pudding (coconut contains a high level of protein)
1 tin coconut milk
2/3 bananas
1 tin of pears/peaches naturally sweetened and drain off liquid
1 passion fruit (optional)

1. Blend all the ingredients in the food processor until a creamy consistency is reached. If a thicker consistency is required, use less coconut milk.

2. Serve chilled in dessert dishes. The mixture may be festively decorated with other fruit, if desired.

Sweet Noodle Pudding a la Ray (Rachael Leader: Fail-Safe Recipes)
½ packet of buckwheat noodles
1 egg (or tablespoon tapioca as egg replacer)
1 small jar of jam, naturally sweetened
4 apples, cored, peeled and grated
2 handfuls raisins or sultanas (unsulphured or organic)
knob of butter

1. Preheat oven to 160°C.

2. In a small bowl, soak raisins or sultanas in boiling water to soften.

3. Meanwhile boil noodles as package directs. Drain.

4. In a mixing bowl, mix jam, lecithin or egg, grated apples, raisins and noodles together. Add the drained noodles and mix through.

5. Lightly grease a square baking dish with olive or avocado oil and place noodle mixture in the dish.

6. Bake for 35 minutes, covered by foil (which does not touch the food). Remove the foil for the last ten minutes.

Baked Apples

Allow 1 apple per person cored sweet cooking apples cold pressed olive
or avocado oil
jam

1. Grease baking dish with olive or avocado oil.

2. Grease apple all over the skin with a little olive or avocado oil,
   just to lubricate.
   Cut the apples in half and take out the pips.

3. Put ½ teaspoon of jam into the centre of each piece of apple. Also, mix a
   dessertspoon of jam into a cup of boiling water and put this into the baking
   dish. Place the apples into this liquid.

4. Cover the dish with foil (do not let the foil touch the apples) and bake at the
   bottom or middle of the oven for 1½ – 2 hours at 160°C, or until soft.

Note

These apples are also delicious when served cold, having been chilled
in the refrigerator.

Fruit Whirl (Optional amounts)

apple
banana
mango
passion fruit
or other fruits (no melon or plums if this recipe accompanies a meal
– they may cause flatulence)

Whirl in a blender or food processor and serve in a festive glass. If eating during
the "protein window period", sprinkle with chopped nuts and seeds (which have
been blended in a food processor). Remember to keep the nuts and seeds in the
refrigerator. ***Exclude cashews and peanuts.***

FESTIVE CAKES AND BISCUITS (DAIRY AND GLUTEN FREE)

Super Cake a la Karen
(Karen Segal)

10 eggs separated and at room temperature
Stevia / Xylitol to taste
6oz dark cooking chocolate melted over hot water and cooled
2 cups finely chopped walnuts (not ground) (optional)

1. Preheat oven to 160°C.

2. Beat the egg yolks and Stevia / Xylitol, until very thick and lemon coloured. Stir in the chocolate and fold in the chopped nuts.

3. Beat the egg whites until stiff but not dry and fold into the chocolate-nut mixture. Put into a greased 10-inch spring form pan and bake for 1 hour or until the centre of the cake springs back when lightly touched with the fingertips. Cool in the pan.

4. A variant could be to use finely grated carrots in place of chocolate.

Chocolate-Chip Biscuits (Gluten Free)
(Janice Trachtman)

200 grams butter
Stevia / Xylitol to taste
2 eggs
2 tsp vanilla essence
1½ cup quinoa
2 cups milk-free chocolate chips
½ cup buckwheat flour
½ cup millet flakes
1 cup desiccated coconut (optional contains protein)
1 tsp gluten free baking soda-bicarbonate (optional)

1. Cream butter, Stevia / Xylitol, vanilla, eggs.

2. Add the dry ingredients and mix thoroughly.

3. Add chocolate chips, coconut and mix.

4. Form into cookies and bake on a greased baking tray for about 10 minutes at 160°C.

Note

Experiment baking these biscuits without the soda-bicarbonate. If absolutely necessary, use the minimum amount.

Almond and Chocolate Cake Delight
250 grams (9oz) chopped almonds
200grams (7oz) dark dairy-free chocolate
Stevia / Xylitol, to taste
7 egg whites
cold pressed olive or avocado oil

1. Blend the almonds, chocolate and Stevia / Xylitol, together in a food processor.

2. Beat egg whites until stiff and fold into the chocolate / almond mixture.

3. Grease a loose bottom cake tin (23cm / 9in) with a little olive or avocado oil and dust with gluten-free flour (corn, buckwheat, potato flour).

4. Put the well mixed mixture into the tin.

5. Bake in the oven at 300°F / 150°C for 1 hour or until firm.

French Chocolate Cake
(Helena Freedman)

4 oz unsalted butter (125 grams)
Stevia / Xylitol, to taste
vanilla essence (a few drops to taste)
6 oz (175 grams) plain cooking chocolate broken into small pieces
1 tsp gluten-free baking powder
2 oz potato flour
4 egg yolks + 4 egg whites

1. Preheat gas oven to mark 4 or electric oven to 160°C. Grease inside of 8 inch round tin with a thin layer of butter.

2. Melt the butter in a saucepan.

3. Add the Stevia / Xylitol, and chocolate pieces to the melted butter and allow to gently dissolve on a low heat, whilst stirring.

4. Remove the saucepan from the hot stove. Beat in the yolks, potato flour and baking powder.

5. In a separate bowl, whisk the egg whites until stiff and then fold gently into the chocolate mixture.

6. When evenly blended, pour the mixture into the prepared baking tin.

7. Bake for approximately 35 minutes. Test with a toothpick.

References

1 Andrew A. Meharg*†, Enzo Lombi‡, Paul N. Williams†, Kirk G. Scheckel§, Joerg Feldmann , Andrea Raab , Yongguan Zhu and Rafiql Islam. January 15, 2008. Speciation and Localization of Arsenic in White and Brown Rice Grains. Environ. Sci. Technol., 2008, 42 (4), pp 1051–1057

Notes:

Chapter 27

Diary Chart Assessment

DATE: .... NAME: .... D.O.B. .... WEIGHT: .... TEL/FAX: ....

TIME notes 24-hour diary	MADOPAR (L-dopa) Dosage and Type	SINEMET (L-dopa) Dosage and Type	Other Drugs, Nutrients and Herbs Dosage (Oral/IV/IM)	Food and Drink Detail	Bowel / Urine	Lifestyle and Emotional Reactions SYMPTOMS	SYMPTOMS Type	SYMPTOMS Time of Relief	SYMPTOMS Time of recurrence
Wake at									
Time									
Time									
Time									
Time									

Chapter 28

Intravenous Nutrition

Intravenous administration of nutrients which are found on biochemical analysis to be deficient in patients, can be more effective than oral supplementation. These, as well as nutrients which play a role in cellular energy production (citric acid cycle) and reduction of oxidative stress (antioxidants), can be administered intravenously. Malabsorption is best supported by this means if the intestinal environment is compromised.

Typical examples of protocols for intravenous nutritional administration are presented below. However, individual physicians will utilise the intravenous nutrients available to them within their own pharmaceutical systems and base their doses on the biochemical individuality of their patients.

Protocol for Intravenous Vitamins and Minerals
by Dr Geoffrey Leader MBChB FRCA

The patient is required to sign informed consent as the effect of administration cannot be predicted with certainty and must be regarded as "nutritional support" and in no way therapeutic. Thereafter, the "cocktail" is dripped slowly into the vein over a period of half an hour, with the patient either in the lying or sitting position, whichever is more comfortable. However, for the first administration, the lying position is always used together with pulse rate and blood pressure monitoring, before, during and after, so as to assess the patient's reactions. Up until the present time, no side effects and especially no allergic reactions have been encountered in a series of 100 administrations.

A typical protocol could include the following vitamins and minerals added to 200ml of sterile water together with heparin 100iu and lignocaine 20mg (to prevent any discomfort), for the average adult.

Ideally the mixture is given twice a week via alternating arm veins. If this is not possible, then they may be given at least once a week, up to a total of eight administrations. After the initial course, a maintenance infusion is usually necessary once a month in order to maintain an in- creased feeling of wellbeing.

However, due to metabolic individuality, some patients may benefit and others not.

Sterile water	200ml	Lignocaine	1% = 2ml
Heparin	100iu	Vits B1 (Thiamine) B2 (Riboflavin) B3 (Niacin)	25 - 50mg 25 - 50mg 25 - 50mg
Vit B12 (Methylcobalamin)	1000mcg	Vit B5 (Dexpanthenol)	500mg
Methylfolate	To be assessed	Magnesium Sulphate	500mg - 1000mg
Vit B6 (Pyridoxine)	25 - 50mg	Molybdenum	50mcg
Zinc	5mg - 10mg	Selenium	80mcg
Chromium	4mcg	Ascorbic acid	1-2gm

Note: Clinical experience of the authors demonstrates that administration of vitamin B6 (pyridoxine) does not present a problem for patients taking L-dopa medication because of the inclusion of decarboxylase inhibitors carbidopa and benserazide respectively in the formulae of "Sinemet" , "Madopar" and "Stalevo". Indeed, vitamin B6 is the necessary co-enzyme with dopa decarboxylase which metabolizes L-dopa to dopamine in the brain. However, both oral and intravenous administration of vitamin B6 should not be concomitant with L-dopa administration but rather when it has already taken effect.

Special Notes Regarding Intravenous Therapy
Each patient needs to be individually assessed to determine suitability and exclude any medical contra indications for intravenous therapy.

The intravenous protocols of Dr Geoffrey Leader are also concomitant within comprehensive oral nutritional and appropriate pharmaceutical support.

Protocol for Intravenous Glutathione
by Dr David Perlmutter MD

There are several factors that explain why glutathione is so beneficial in Parkinson's disease. Glutathione has the unique ability to make certain areas of the brain more sensitive to dopamine[1], so that even though dopamine is decreased, it nevertheless becomes more effective. The concept of enhancing cellular receptor sensitivity has become quite familiar in medicine today. In diabetes for example, before actually administering insulin, physicians often begin therapy by prescribing the drug metformin, which acts by enhancing the sensitivity of cells to whatever insulin is still being produced.

My protocol for using glutathione is relatively simple. Glutathione is inexpensive and easily obtained. I use liquid glutathione, not reconstituted powder. It should be administered by a medical practitioner as follows:

1. Dilute the appropriate dosage of glutathione liquid in 10cc of sterile normal saline. Usually vials contain 200mg.

2. This solution is then injected through a 21-gauge butterfly catheter intravenously over a 15 to 20 minute period of time.

3. Alternatively, many patients choose to have an intravenous access port inserted. This allows frequent glutathione administration without repeated intravenous injections. Treatment begins at 1000mg glutathione 3 times a week but dosage and frequency may be further adjusted depending on response.

The Importance of Glutathione
With so much emphasis placed on L-dopa therapy, it is important to recognise that another vital brain chemical is also profoundly deficient in Parkinson's disease. This chemical, glutathione, is substantially reduced, virtually across the board, in Parkinson's patients. And yet, this deficiency seems to receive precious little attention[2]. Glutathione is a critically important brain chemical. It is clearly one of the most important brain antioxidants. That is, glutathione helps to preserve brain tissue by reducing damage from free radicals[3] - destructive chemicals formed by the normal processes of metabolism, toxic elements in the environment, and as a normal response of the body to challenges by infectious agents or other stresses. In addition to quenching dangerous free radicals, glutathione also acts to recycle vitamin C and vitamin E, which, because of their antioxidant activity, also reduce free radicals in the brain. The Department of Neurology, University of Sassari, Italy conducted a study with glutathione administration. In this research protocol, Parkinson's patients received intravenous glutathione twice daily for 30 days. The subjects were then evaluated at one month intervals for up to six months. The published results indicated "all patients improved significantly after glutathione therapy, with a 42% decline in disability.

Once glutathione was stopped the therapeutic effect lasted 2-4 months." Further, the researchers indicated "...glutathione has symptomatic efficacy and possibly retards the progression of the disease"[4]. This Italian study demonstrated that providing glutathione, a substance naturally occurring in the brain, provided Parkinson's patients with substantial benefit.

Special Note Regarding Intravenous Therapy
Each patient needs to be individually assessed to determine suitability and exclude any medical contra indications for intravenous therapy.

References

1. SS Oja, R Jankay, V Varga, P Saransaari: 2000: Modulation of Glutamate Receptor Functions by Glutathione: Neurochem Int Aug-Sept 37 (2-3): pps. 299-306

2. T L Perry, D V Godin, S Hansen: 1982: Parkinson's Disease - A disorder due to nigral glutathione deficiency?: Neurosci Lett 33: pps. 305-310

3. B H Juurlin, P G Paterson: 1998: Review of oxidative stress in brain and spinal cord injury: Suggestions for pharmacological and nutritional management strategies: J Spinal Cord Med Oct: 21 (4): pps. 309-334

4. G Sechi, M G Deledda, G Bua, et al: 1996: Reduced Glutathione in the treatment of early Parkinson's Disease: Prog Neuropsychopharmacol Biol Psychiatry 20(7): pps. 1159-70

Notes:

Chapter 29

Undergoing Anaesthesia
Nutritional Considerations

1. Two weeks before surgery (if possible), cease taking nutrients which affect the clotting potential of the blood. These include vitamin C and vitamin E as well as Omega 6 (GLA) and Omega 3 (EPA) (Essential Fatty Acids).

   There are also medicinal herbs which thin the blood. These should be omitted together with the above nutrients well before the date of surgery. It is important to check the properties of nutrients and herbs and the interactions between them and with drugs.

2. Ensure good bowel function before surgery. If constipation is a problem, 2-3 pre-soaked prunes taken between meals over the day may be helpful. 8 – 10 glasses of water sipped over the day and Caricol (papaya extract) taken with main meals. The GP should be consulted if constipation remains a problem prior to surgery.

3. For five days prior to surgery red meat should be avoided. This requires a great deal of digestion and has a longer transit time through the gut than other proteins such as fish and the white of chicken (no skin.) Alcohol should be avoided and caffeine-containing food and drinks should be reduced (tea, coffee, chocolate.)

4. Four hours before surgery a drink can be taken – ½ a glass of still, clear unsweetened apple juice, diluted with ½ a glass of still mineral water. Anaesthesiologists find that it is important to maintain blood sugar levels and fluid prior to surgery, and this fluid will have passed out of the stomach well before actual surgery if taken strictly four hours before. In special pathological circumstances, the time of pre-surgical nutritional support may be reduced at the discretion of the individual anaesthesiologists[1, 2.]

5. After surgery, it is most suitable to replace the first meal with a **pre-digested** elemental food. This is more easily and quickly absorbed than solid food and therefore is more appropriate after surgery as digestion is not optimal at this time.

6. Administration of vitamins C and E, Essential Fatty Acids - Omega 6 and Omega 3, or any medicinal herbs which affect platelet aggregation (clotting factors) should only be resumed after wound-healing is established. There is no contraindication, however, for probiotics and saccharomyces boulardi which are helpful for optimisation of gut immunity.

7. Regulation of bowel function after surgery can be a problem due to analgesic medication or other reasons. When allowed, taking 8 – 10 cups of fluid daily is essential and 2-3 pre-soaked prunes eaten at intervals over the day between meals as well as Caricol (papaya extract) can be helpful. It is important to speak to the medical team about possible preventive action such as taking a mild laxative daily until normal intestinal movement can be re-established.

The authors cannot take responsibility for post–operative recommendations for regulation of bowel function.

8. Dopaminergic drugs can be taken with a very small sip of water prior to surgery and post-operatively. However this must be authorised by the attendant anaesthesiologist. A patient should arrange consultation with the anaesthesiologist before the day of surgery. Drugs used in anaesthesia may interact with your medication.

9. It is also very important to record the exact times when your drugs are due so that these can be replicated as far as possible in hospital. If time permits, it will be helpful to have your medication changed from Sinemet to Madopar Dispersible which is more quickly absorbed and can also be given by naso-gastric tube directly into the stomach if necessary. It is necessary for a trial of Madopar Dispersible well before surgery date to check whether it is well tolerated.

Post–operatively

■ Ensure early mobilisation and breathing exercises, especially where there is stiffness of the chest wall, so as to help to prevent deep vein thrombosis and atelectasis (collapse of the lungs.) It would be prudent to ask for physiotherapy at the time of consultation with the anaesthetist.

■ When sitting up from the lying position do so slowly so as to avoid dizziness which can be related to your condition.

■ Peppermint tea and ginger root tea may be helpful for nausea. However, anti-emetic drugs may also be indicated, excluding Metoclopramide, Phenothiazines and Butyrophenones.

■ It is essential to restart your medication as soon as possible with sips of water.

■ At the end of anaesthesia an infusion of low dose B vitamins, glutathione and very low dose of vitamin C may help to aid detoxification of anaesthetic drugs and speed up recovery from anaesthesia[3].

■ It may also be prudent to add other anti-oxidant nutrients to the infusion, as mentioned below. This concept of **very gently** enhancing detoxification is an important one for general anaesthesia and particularly in Parkinson's Disease patients. This is because of the possibly compromised cytochrome P450 liver detoxification pathway.[4, 5, 6]

■ Analgesics may cause constipation. Appropriate diet, fluids and laxatives may need to be prescribed (see above protocol).

Gentle Natural Detoxification

by Helen Kimber BSc (Hons) PGCE ECNP

General guidelines

Vitamin C, the B vitamins and bioflavonoids all contribute to the activity of the cytochrome P450 enzyme system[7] which may be compromised in Parkinson's Disease. These nutrients are also extremely powerful antioxidants. They work in conjunction with vitamin E to quench free radical processes which arise from the detoxification reactions of the liver.

High quality protein foods are rich sources of glutathione as well as the sulphur amino acid cysteine. Glutathione helps to regulate phase II conjugation reactions[8].

Dedicated intense detoxification regimes are not suitable for Parkinson's Disease patients.

Nutritional support must always be under the supervision of healthcare professionals.

References

1. Erskine L, Hunt JN: 1981: The gastric emptying of small volumes given in quick succession: J Physiol: 313: pps. 334-35

2. Brener W, Hendrix TR, McHugh R: 1983: Regulation of the gastric emptying of glucose: Gastroenterology: 85: pps. 76-82

3. Anderson KE, Kappas: 1991: A Dietary Regulation of cytochrome P450: Annual Review of Nutrition Vol. 11: pps. 141-67

4. C M Tanner: 1991: Abnormal Liver Enzyme-mediated Metabolism in Parkinson's Disease - A Second Look: Neurology 41: (5 suppl 2): pps. 89-92

5. S Williams, A Sturman, G Steventon, R Waring: 1991: Metabolic Biomarkers of Parkinson's Disease: Acta Neurologica Scandinavica: Supplementum 136: pps. 19-23

6. Liver Enzyme Abnormalities in Parkinson's Disease: 1991: Geriatrics 46 Suppl 1: pps. 60-63

7. Anderson KE, Kappas: 1991: A Dietary Regulation of cytochrome P450: Annual Review of Nutrition Vol. 11: pps. 141-67

8. Beutler E: 1989: Nutritional and Metabolic Aspects of Glutathione: Annual Review of Nutrition Vol 9: pps. 287-302

Chapter 30

Dental Health

Dental and oral health are vital considerations. Teeth are used for chewing, during which salivary amylase is produced to facilitate digestion and the oral cavity influences speech and articulation.

There are many research papers published in prestigious, peer- reviewed journals on the subject of mercury – a large number with particular reference to mercury amalgam fillings and toxicity. There are some studies which are pertinent to people with Parkinson's disease[1]. Although the studies referenced in this chapter are related to Parkinson's disease, the issue of mercury toxicity remains contentious.

Mercury accumulates in brain tissue and affects the central nervous system. When combined with a measurable electrical current (the battery effect) of dental fillings, it would be expected that there would be some changes in brain activity – itself an electrical organ – when measured by EEG. This is indeed so[2, 3].

Toxic levels of fluoride may be ingested. This should be monitored where possible. Besides sodium fluoride in toothpaste, fluoride content is increasing in our food due to the heavy reliance on fertilisers, which are rich in fluoride as well as fluoridated drinking water. Dental fluorosis or mottled teeth can be an indication of fluoride poisoning.

Research has demonstrated medical concerns associated with sodium fluoride (United States National Research Council 2006).

Recommendations

- Regular visits to a Dental Hygienist / Dentist for cleaning of the teeth, assessment of the gums and monitoring.

- Dentures should be well fitting.

- *Non-mercury* amalgam should be used for fillings[4].

- If mercury fillings are removed, this should be done by a Dentist who is familiar with Chelation Therapy for mercury and the safety procedures during mercury removal. **However, it is important for Parkinson's people**

not to have all their mercury fillings removed at one time, as detoxification can be a problem. Great care must be given to the decision to remove mercury fillings.
Advice can be obtained from a dentist who practices specialized safe mercury removal and dentistry, with all its implications.

- If cleaning manually is difficult, an electric toothbrush may be easier. Assistance may be needed for control of brushing.

- Fluoride levels should be monitored. The acknowledged safety limit is 3mg of fluoride a day[5].

- Assessment by the dentist of the temporomandibular joint (TMJ). Attention should be paid to the alignment of the TMJ as if it is mal-aligned it may become a stressor, affecting posture and Parkinson's symptoms.

Dr. John Beck M.D, orthopaedic surgeon in the United States has explained that the brain receives 40% of its information about posture from the soles of the feet, 40% from the position of the mandible and 20% from the spine. To quote Dr. Beck: "The brain is sensitive to the neuroposture being off by as little as 1 millimetre from the line of gravity."

References

1. Herrero PY: 1983: Mercury- Chronic Poisoning in Encyclopaedia of Occ. Health and Safety: 3rd Edition, Vol. 2: Int. Labour Office, Geneva: pps. 1334-1335

2. Popov L, Gig T, Prof Zabol: 1973: Bioelec. Activity of the Brain in Patients with Chronic Occupational Mercury Poisoning: Russian BCC J.17: p. 52

3. Piikivi, Tolonen U: 1989: EEG Findings in Chlor. Alkali Workers Subjected to Low Long Term Exposure to Mercury Vapour: Brit J Industrial Medicine 46: p. 370

4. British Society for Mercury Free Dentistry: 225 Old Brompton Road, London, SW5 0EA, UK: Tel. +44 (20) 8746 1177

5. McDonagh MS, Whiting PF, Wilson PM, Sutton AJ, Chestnutt I, Cooper J, Misso K, Bradley M, Treasure E, Kleijnen J: 2000: Systematic review of water fluoridation: British Medical Journal 7: pps. 844-5

Bibliography

United States National Research Council
Mercury in Dentistry: 2006: Dr Jack Levenson
Parkinson's Disease – The Way Forward! An Integrated Approach including Drugs, Surgery, Nutrition, Bowel and Muscle Function, Self-Esteem, Sexuality, Stress Control and Carers: Dr Geoffrey Leader and Lucille Leader with Contributions by Prof Aroldo Rossi, Dr Lia Rossi-Prosperi et al. and Foreword by Prof Leslie Findley (Denor Press)

Chapter 31

Stress
The Dopamine Connection!

Many people with Parkinson's Disease find that their symptoms of motor disturbance are exacerbated by stress. This is not surprising when one realizes that adrenaline, the hormone released in response to stress, is metabolized from dopamine! Feedback from adrenaline compromises the production of L-dopa (catecholamine feedback inhibits tyrosine hydroxylase[1]). Stress also affects gastrointestinal function, pH levels, glycaemic control, cortisol elevation and the immune system!

Depression and stress often affect people with Parkinson's Disease. This can be due to the illness itself as dopamine metabolises (is converted) to noradrenaline and adrenaline. However, it would be unnatural if people were not feeling depressed at having developed this illness.

Therefore, in order to reduce stress-related symptoms, it is vital for patients to have strong medical and psychological support as well as engaging in activities which offer deep mind-body relaxation and the release of excess emotional charge.

Stress appears in many ways!
- Psychological pain which is still carried from the past

- Acute psychological pain associated with present situations

- Worry about Parkinson's Disease and the consequences

- Interpersonal changes in relationships and lifestyle due to the onset of illness

- Sexual problems

- Concerns about the wellbeing of partners and care givers

- Physical pain

- Fear of "freezing", problems with getting up, sitting down, turning over in bed, walking

- Fear of incontinence, constipation, diarrhoea

- Nervousness, stress and apprehension associated with daily activities or demands

- Illness (e.g. a cold, virus, infection, other illness) other than Parkinson's Disease

- Temporomandibular Joint (TMJ) related problems

- Having to move at an inappropriate speed

- Medications (medical or street drugs)

- Surgery

- Anaesthesia

- Worry about food purchase, preparation

- Chewing and swallowing problems

- Food intolerances / allergy

- Chemical sensitivities

- Financial concerns

Therapists

Experience demonstrates that people who have supportive therapy and counseling cope best with their stress-related symptoms. The following health professionals may be helpful:

- Clinical Psychologist – to identify areas of stress and counseling

- Psychiatrist – if medically indicated

- Hypnotherapist – to release emotional charge, to achieve / learn relaxation and to address emotional / psychological issues that may affect patients and cause unnecessary stress

- Autogenic Training – to teach techniques to achieve deep mind-body relaxation. It offers invaluable tools for symptom control as well as the lowering of blood pressure and heart rate. It can be of benefit to patients / partners and care givers

- Movement Therapist – to help with movement problems including "freezing", balance, walking and changing of positions

- Occupational Therapist – to organize movement, special aids (bath, beds, chairs, utensils etc)

- Physiotherapist, Osteopath - to assist with musculo-skeletal health, movement facilitation and pain relief

- Biofeedback Therapist – to enable patients to monitor muscle tension so that relaxation techniques can be implemented

- Tai Chi Teacher – for relaxation, balance training and circulation

- Masseur / Masseuse – to relieve tension and muscle spasm and improve circulation

- Speech Therapist – to maintain speech and swallowing functions

- Sexual Therapist – for adaptation and reassurance

- Incontinence Nurses

- Nutritionist - to assist with food compatible with L-dopa, bowel function, mitochondrial energy stimulation, adrenal support, chewing and swallowing problems, diet and weight management

- Dentist and Dental Hygienist – to maintain mouth hygiene and good fitting dentures

- Music Therapist, Art Therapist, Dance Therapist – for emotional release and co-ordination

- Relaxing hobbies – for wellbeing

- Meditation, Mindfulness, Belief / Religious Faith (for some) – for the soul

See over for other helpful recommendations ➡

Other helpful recommendations

- Exercising / walking

- Singing

- Laughter therapy (comedy videos, joke books,) avoiding depressing subjects

- Attending entertainment

- Visiting friends / inviting guests

- Bathing in a whirlpool or jacuzzi (always with someone present).

- Avoiding kitchen stress: have liquids prepared in thermos flasks - especially easy are those with a pump mechanism. Straws will make drinking easier and less stressful. Occupational Therapists can direct patients to specialized utensils, which may be easier to use and control. If people are on their own, buying and preparing food can be stressful, especially if movement is difficult. The General Practitioner may well be able to recommend organizations, which can help. Delivery of ready-made foods from shops is also a possibility. If movement and safety are problems, a microwave oven may need to be used. As microwave ovens carry their own health risks, using this form of cooking is only for emergencies or movement problems.

- Learning techniques for getting out of and turning in bed: silk sheets and pyjamas facilitate turning.

- Getting up in the morning: physiotherapist/movement therapist can provide stretching, toning, mobilizing and breathing exercises to be done in bed before getting up, to increase circulation/reduce stiffness. Hypnotherapy/autogenic training techniques before rising are helpful.

- Bathing and Showering: Warm water helps with muscle relaxation, circulation and a feeling of wellbeing. If lying is a problem, a "walk- in" type of "sitting-bath" bath is available. Shower cubicles can be supplied with seats.

- Hydrotherapy: Movement is facilitated when limbs are supported by warm water. Referral is to a physiotherapist for hydrotherapy and specialized exercises (done in a warm hydrotherapy pool).

Stress and Nutritional Support

Adrenal Stress Index Test (Saliva)[2]
Cortisol may be elevated due to stress. This test is a measure of cortisol and DHEA levels and is used as a biochemical marker of stress. Alteration of the levels of these hormones may have beneficial therapeutic effects.

Adrenal Support
Vitamin C, Vitamin B5 and Vitamin B Complex are important in adrenal function. (see chapter 7, page 21 for recommendations). Panax and Siberian ginseng have also been shown to be helpful.

Blood Sugar Balance
Stress influences the concentration of glucose (blood sugar) in the blood. The concentration of blood glucose then increases and Parkinson's People often note that stress indeed exacerbates their movement disturbance. In order to maintain more control over blood sugar levels, stress control and diet management protocols are vital.

A well-timed appropriate diet is helpful whether people are on L-dopa drugs or not.

- Eating three main meals daily. Remember that four hours after eating, glucose from the previous meal has been absorbed. Glucose is the necessary "fuel source for cell energy production and consequently other functions, including dopamine metabolism.

- Eating a small snack every two hours (between meals) may help maintain an even blood sugar level. Snacks should contain small portions of complex carbohydrates (an apple / apple sauce or soup containing sweet potato with other vegetables). Add a ½ teaspoon of organic coconut oil to the snack as this can be used as an alternative fuel sauce to glucose which in some cases may not be optimally used in Parkinson's Disease.

  Almonds and other nuts (not peanuts or cashews which may contain mycotoxins), together with fruit, are a good combination.

  Use nuts or seeds in powdered form if swallowing or chewing are a possible problem. **Users of L-dopa need to be aware of the protein – L-dopa interaction (nuts contain a predominant amount of protein) and can only use this combination during a "protein window".**

- Gradually reduce sweets and sugary foods, refined carbohydrates, alcohol and caffeine. Substitute these with healthy delicious alter- natives including herb teas, fruit and fruit juices (dilute 50% water), toast and crackers with hummus, tahini, almond and other spreads.

- Adding a little unheated oil, such as cold pressed olive or avocado oil to a glucose rich meal or snack may be helpful in that glucose release will be slowed down resulting in subtle longer sustained energy. (Never heat polyunsaturated oils or they become dangerous trans fats. Olive or avocado oil may be heated but not above 160°C as this will result in the production of trans fats).

- If indicated medically, glucomannan fibre[3] can be taken as a supplement. This is a complex carbohydrate fibre, which is effective in stabilizing blood sugar levels. However, the effect of this fibre on L-dopa ("Stalevo", "Sinemet", "Madopar" or equivalent drug) needs to be assessed individually as the protein portion, although small, may compete at the absorption sites with L-dopa and undermine its effects.

- Nutritional biochemical testing assesses the status of vitamins and minerals involved in the regulation of blood sugar. Deficiencies need supplementing.

References

1. Victor W. Rodwell, David A. Bender et al: 2015: Harper's Illustrated Biochemistry 30th Edition: McGraw Hill Education, USA: Biosynthesis of Catecholamines p. 509

2. Great Smokies Diagnostic Laboratory, Ashville, North Carolina, USA: UK rep: Nutri Ltd: +44 (0)800 212 742

3. Patrick Holford BSc Dip ION: 1992: Optimum Nutrition Workbook: ION Press, London, UK: p.148

Note:

1. The British Autogenic Society, London, WC1N 3HR Website: www.autogenic-therapy.org.uk

2. Galin Tudhope BA Psych MSc LCD Dip AT (Autogenic Training/ Psychotherapy) Email: Gaylin@5tconsulting.net

3. David Uri DHP FAPHP MNCH NGH(USA) FRSH Email: davideuri@yahoo.co.uk
   Parkinson's Disease – Relaxation (CD Recording)
   ISBN - 10: 0-9551661-0-1   ISBN - 13: 978-0-9551661-0-5
   Order: Nutri Centre UK Tel: +44 (0)20 73232382 / Shops / Amazon

Psychologists and other healthcare professionals may be accessed through the Medical Practitioner.

Chapter 32

Improving Sleep

Some people have difficulty in falling asleep or awaken during the night, finding it difficult to sleep again. There are many reasons for sleep difficulties and REM sleep can be significantly reduced[1] in Parkinson's Disease. This chapter, however, will only address the practical and nutritional aspects.

Practical Strategies

- One should wind down physically and mentally after the evening meal. It is necessary to be as physically and mentally relaxed as possible before switching off the light and going to sleep. Light reading is relaxing.
- Autogenic Training techniques (Note1) when in bed, provide excellent tools for deep mind-body relaxation. Listening to a dedicated relaxation recording, such as Parkinson's Disease Relaxation (Note 2), in bed, is helpful.
- In the evening, refrain from using electronic devices, including televisions, mobile phones, tablets, PC's. They emit blue light, which affects the production of the hormone Melatonin (which is necessary for sleep). Bright light also has this effect. Wearing blue light blocking glasses and exposing oneself to dim rather than bright light in the evening, could be helpful[2,3]. Melatonin can be medically prescribed if indicated.
- Research studies have indicated that exposure to 'Pink Noise' has been found to improve the restorative phase of sleep called 'slow wave sleep'. Technology is available to provide this sound to encourage and support sleep.
- No light should shine into the room. It disrupts melatonin production.
- Room temperature should be comfortably warm / cool, bed coverings not too heavy / light, pillows filling the space between head and shoulder and mattress in good condition. Be aware of any sensitivity to any materials used, including soap powder.
- Silk sheets and pyjamas facilitate movement. "Controlled Release (CR)" L dopa can be helpful at night but be aware of the protein-drug "window".
- If pain is a problem, a physiotherapist will recommend optimum body position for lying and techniques for safely getting in and out of bed. An occupational therapist can also provide helpful aids.
- Sometimes, an "intracellular calcium block" in Parkinson's may contribute to muscle spasm. Discuss possible magnesium supplementation with the medical doctor and clinical nutritionist (Test: Magnesium red cell status).

- Empty bladder or bowels before going to bed. If sleep is disrupted by the need for toilet use, acquire a commode to keep by the bed, especially if stability is a problem. Medical review is always necessary if there are urinary or intestinal problems.

Nutritional Strategies

- Ensure fluids are not consumed after 6pm. However, it is important to drink sufficient fluid during the day, to ensure optimal bowel and urinary function.
- Ensure that no caffeine-containing drinks or foods (coffee, chocolate, teas except for camomile) have been taken for some hours before going to bed. If "Controlled Release (CR)" L-dopa has been taken at night, dense protein foods should be avoided until wear-off.
- Heavy evening meals after 6pm should be avoided. Digestion at night can be a problem.
- Eating a small portion of apple sauce with a little mashed banana or having a little vegetable (include sweet potato) soup before sleep, may support blood sugar levels. The brain uses up its energy fuel every four hours and it is important that if one wakes during the night, eating one of these snacks before returning to bed as may be beneficial. It could be that blood sugar levels have dropped and this is one of the possible reasons for sleep disturbance.
- Autogenic Training (Note 1) techniques or a specialized relaxing recording (Note 2), may be helpful.

If all fails, it is best to get out of bed, snack, read, watch television, listen to the radio or indulge in some absorbing activity! People find that they will usually sleep when they are truly tired enough!

References

1. Apps MC, Sheaff PC et al: 1985: Respiration and Sleep in Parkinson's Disease: Journal of Neurology, Neurosurgery and Psychiatry: Vol 48: pps. 1240-1245
2. Wood B1, Rea MS, Plitnick B, Figueiro MG: Epub 2012 Jul 31: Light level and duration of exposure determine the impact of self-luminous tablets on melatonin suppression: Appl Ergon. 2013 Mar;44(2): 237-40. doi: 10.1016/j.apergo.2012.07.008
3. Wood B1, Rea MS, Plitnick B, Figueiro MG: Applied Ergonomics: Volume 44, Issue 2, March 2013, Light level and duration of exposure determine the impact of self-luminous tablets on melatonin suppression: Pages 237–240, http://dx.doi.org/10.1016/j.apergo.2012.07.008

Note:

1. British Autogenic Society, London, UK
2. Parkinson's Disease Relaxation by David Uri (CD Recording)
   ISBN10: 0-9551661-0-1 ISBN13: 978-0-9551661-0-5

Chapter 33

Sexuality

Nutritional Aspects

William Shakespeare wrote in his wonderful sonnet, *True Love:*

> *... Love is not love*
> *which alters when it alteration finds, Or bends with the*
> *remover to remove. O no! it is an ever-fixed mark*
> *that looks on tempests, and is never shaken ...*

Both partners in the relationship need confirmation that their emotional attachment or love for each other remains untouched by any impediment or handicap.

In some cases, people who develop a movement disorder, such as Parkinson's Disease, are embarrassed by their movement disturbance – and so they withdraw! This is not because their feelings for their partners have waned. Sometimes, it is because they doubt their partners' continued feelings for them, in view of new mental, physical, practical and emotional adjustments that may be necessary.

This doubt can cause their healthy partners to feel rejected, wrongly believing that their affected partner is not capable of "feeling" for them anymore. The consequences are tragic and easily avoided if partners communicate honestly with each other and if necessary, seek the advice of a sexual therapist or counsellor.

> **The correct mindset is essential!**
> **Whenever you feel like taking *one* step backwards,**
> **take *two* forwards!**

Apart from sexual intercourse and outercourse[1] (intimacy without penetration), there are other successful ways to give personal assurances of one's continued recognition and affection – regular hugs and words of love work wonders for the soul as do words of praise and appreciation, little gifts and cards, arranging an outing or holiday and individual "space" for both partners.

Maintaining interest in appearance and personal hygiene (regular shower/bath, attention to teeth, face, hair, nails, clothes) is important for the self-esteem of both partners. It promotes continued mutual in- terest and admiration.

> Love is like a rose – to remain in bloom,
> it requires watering, daily...
>
> Always keep a sense of humor!
>
> Imagine yourself "in the shoes" of your partner...
>
> If you need help, ask your doctor to refer you to the appropriate specialist
>
> Try not to worry unnecessarily – assistance is available!

Intimacy
Practical Nutritional Considerations

- Don't be tired! Don't be hungry!

   For a feeling of wellbeing and support of energy and blood sugar levels, the daily diet should be well balanced (and appropriate to the drug regime). Taking a small snack every two hours, which contains a complex carbohydrate, can often help to regulate blood sugar levels and support general energy. Vegetable soup containing green vegetables and sweet potatoes and apple puree are light and energizing.

- A light meal only!

   A *heavy meal* is inappropriate before intimacy as it may cause sluggishness or bloating. Some people also find that a heavy meal compromises the absorption and efficacy of their L-dopa.

- Alcohol can be a "downer!"

   Although relaxing, alcohol may possibly dull the senses and affect balance. It has been recommended that it be avoided by those who take centrally acting medication[2.]

■ Wait until L-dopa is working!

If one is taking L-dopa medication, it is best to wait until it "kicks in" before physical expression. ***"Madopar" Dispersible often kicks-in more quickly than capsules or tablets.*** It would be prudent to discuss using this form of L-dopa with the attendant doctor.

■ Watch out for drug-nutrient interaction!

If food is to be eaten around the time of intimacy, only foods that are compatible with L-dopa absorption should be eaten. The following scheme might be helpful:

a) Take L-dopa.

b) Wait until the drug has "kicked in" and only then eat very *lightly* – some *fruit or vegetables or vegetable soup* (no grapefruit, avocado, asparagus, pulses, soy, nuts, seeds, animal produce, dairy, wheat, couscous, kamut, bulgar, sago, rye, oats, barley, spelt). In this context, something light is far better than a meal containing dense protein.

■ Avoid constipation!

Maintaining regular daily bowel movement is essential for a feeling of wellbeing as well as for the optimum absorption of drugs.

■ Remember to empty your bladder!

This is essential preparation for comfort during intimacy.

■ Any low-fat diet followed should not exclude the Essential Fatty Acids (Omega 6 and Omega 3) found in seeds and nuts (exclude peanuts and cashews as they might contain mycotoxins) – and oily fish such as herring, sardines, mackerel and salmon. As cholesterol is the precursor of male and female hormones (oestrogen, progesterone and testosterone), it should not be allowed to fall below the normal range.

- Some nutritional deficiencies can compromise energy production[3] as can some drugs. Examples of nutrients which may be deficient and which are used in cells to manufacture energy, include CoQ10, B vitamins, vitamin C, iron and copper. Nutritional status should be assessed by biochemical tests and any deficiencies demonstrated should be addressed. Iron is only ever supplemented if found to be a cellular deficiency. However it is vital to note that iron may only be supplemented as subject to laboratory demonstration of cellular deficiency.

- Anti-oxidant therapy may be prudent if Sildenafil (Viagra) is taken as this drug enhances nitric oxide production[4] and increases free radical production. Antioxidants include Vitamins C and E, selenium and alpha - lipoic acid. Glutathione is also an antioxidant. It is best-administered intravenously. However, it can also be taken orally in the form of its precursor, n-acetyl cysteine, in low doses.

- Zinc is implicated in male sexual function. However, nutrients should only be taken under professional supervision. There are other forms of management (nutritional, herbal or pharmaceutical) which should only be prescribed by a medical practitioner.

References

1. Gila Bronner MPH MSW, Head of Sex Therapy Service, Sexual Medicine Centre, Department of Urology, Sheba Medical Centre, Class-Clinic, Tel Hashomer, Israel: Email: gilab@netvision.net.il

2. ABPI Compendium of Data Sheets and Summaries of Product Characteristics (1999-2000): Datapharm Publications Ltd, London, UK: p. 1610

3. Lucille Leader: Optimising Function by Nutritional Manipulation - Energy Production: In Dr Geoffrey Leader, Lucille Leader, et al: 2006: Parkinson's Disease - The Way Forward!: Denor Press, London, UK: p. 79

4. Dr David Perlmutter MD: 2000: BrainRecovery.Com: Perlmutter Health Center, Naples, FL, USA: p. 26

Bibliography

Dr Michael Perring: 2006: Sexuality in Parkinson's Disease: In Dr Geoffrey Leader, Lucille Leader, et al: Parkinson's Disease - The Way Forward!: Denor Press, London, UK

Gila Bronner, Vladimir Royter, Amos Korczyn, Nir Giladi: 2004: Sexual Dysfunction in Parkinson's Disease: Journal of Sex & Marital Therapy: Vol 30

Gila Bronner, Vladimir Royter, Amos Korczyn, Nir Giladi: 2003: Sexuality and Parkinson's Disease: In Edited by M-A Bedard et al: Mental and Behavioural Dysfunction in Movement Disorders: Humana Press Inc., Totowa, NJ, USA

Chapter 34

The Carers' Guide

Caregivers should always maintain a sense of great self-worth as human beings and as pivotal members of the Parkinson's Disease Management Team. Without the full collaboration of Caregivers, the "team" effort would fail to provide optimum support of the Parkinson's Disease patient.

There is nothing more distressing than the feeling of helplessness arising from not knowing how to help manage the general daily functional health of the person with Parkinson's Disease (PD).

Eating and bowel function are underlying necessities for life and wellbeing. In Parkinson's Disease there are specific guidelines which can be helpful in optimizing these functions which are often so compromised in those suffering from PD.

The chapters in this book are presented in an easy-to-follow, user- friendly style. The authors are aware that it is mainly the Caregivers who will offer "wrap-around care" to their charges. The authors offer solutions which are helpful tools to equip the Caregiver to deal with these vital necessities of functional health for the person living with PD. These include knowing:

- which foods will not interfere with the absorption and efficacy of L-dopa

- when to eat in order to help reduce dyskinesia

- when to eat in order to avoid drug-related nausea

- which foods and fluids facilitate bowel movement

- simple and delicious recipes which are compatible with L-dopa absorption *yet suitable for the whole family*

- which foods contain important vitamins, minerals and essential fatty acids

- how to use basic charts to assess the most appropriate dosage of drugs, the "kick-in" and efficacy times of L-dopa, in order to smooth out the "on-off" discomfort

- how to improve the possibilities for intimacy

Caring for a loved one at home is a very demanding vocation. Watching someone suffering physically, mentally and emotionally can be very draining. Due to the illness of one family member, there may be a need for an exchange of roles within the family unit. For instance, someone who has previously been "cared for" will now have to become the "active caregiver". This is a very difficult adaptation and spouses and partners would be well advised to seek the support of a professional counsellor to guide them with the necessary realignment of the cornerstones of their lives.

Caregivers also have personal rights! They often tend to forget this in their constant devotion. Caregivers, sometimes impulsively out of goodwill, carry out tasks unnecessarily for their charges which are still within the capability of the patient. This can easily lead to an "unreasonably" dependent attitude. This situation should be avoided at all costs, both in the interests of the patient's self-esteem as well as for the Caregiver, and should be sensitively negotiated between both parties.

Whether the care is given on a personal or professional level, Caregivers must care for themselves physically, mentally and emotionally if they are to remain stable, well and capable of empathetic support to the best of their ability. Frustrated and exhausted people cannot provide the best environment for themselves or for patients.

Caregivers can become increasingly socially isolated by their own devotion to their charge. Within a partnership or a family setting, if a Caregiver becomes ill as a result of the emotional and physical demands of caring, there may be no-one to look after the Caregiver or the ill person! With this in mind, it is certainly not selfish for Caregivers of any age to preciously guard their own health and wellbeing – in fact it is essential in order to remain an Optimum Caregiver!

Regular respite care should be organised so that caregivers can have time and space to relax and regain physical and emotional energy, to exercise, follow interests and have social contact which may be difficult if those they care for are very ill. Outings could include visits to cultural and other events, as well as appointments with counsellors for support and guidance. Such breaks from routine can assist in restoring vitality and will lift the Caregiver's mood so that he/she will be able to express loving care in a more relaxed way. *If, however, there is no possibility of relief due to practical or financial circumstances, perhaps local community or religious centres could be approached as these groups can frequently offer voluntary assistance.*

Very dependent patients are usually difficult to placate, as they are genuinely afraid that no one else is as trustworthy as their own family or close friend. It is imperative, however, for healthy family members to maintain balanced contact outside the home where they can move and express themselves freely. Caregivers need to express their needs, gently but firmly to those for whom they care, whilst reaffirming their love and concern. In some cases, asking the ill person to imagine a reversal of roles with the Caregiver might help in providing a more accepting and tolerant attitude in very difficult situations.

It is quite understandable that Caregivers should feel frustrated and disappointed at life's circumstances. Healthcare professionals do observe this in some instances in the clinic where partners present together. Caregivers need counselling to enable them to express their anger, fear or other emotions. "Bottling up" such feelings of resentment can result in them unconsciously "taking it out" on their charges (for instance caregivers expressing impatience with the patient's disability in the presence of a third party). This causes excruciating humiliation to patients. Whilst this is understandable because of the unremitting stress and frustration experienced, it demonstrates that all good intentions can easily be undermined if well-meaning and devoted Caregivers remain unsupported and become emotionally exhausted.

Caregivers should not lose pride in their physical appearance and presentation - weight, hair, nails, face and clothes. This is essential for their self-esteem and their loving relationship with an ill partner. The person with Parkinson's Disease is still capable of appreciating an attractive appearance!

There are support groups for Caregivers. Parkinson's Disease Societies should be able to direct Caregivers to these groups. Counsellors can usually be recommended by a Caregiver's doctor. Religious and community centres are to be found in most areas.

Some personal recommendations for Caregivers

- Count the blessings that you still have and appreciate yourself as a worthy and loving human being who is capable of a very special job of very special deeds

- Autogenic Training/Hypnotherapy sessions for deep mind and body relaxation

- Dancing Classes / Gym / Swimming

- Playing a musical instrument/Music Therapy

- Joining a library

- Joining a religious affiliation, if so inclined

- Yoga, Qi Gong or Tai Chi exercise classes

- Cinema / Shows / Concerts

- Group therapy

- Counselling

- Keeping social contact and regularly inviting friends / family

- Enjoy a laugh each day - rent a comedy video, acquire a book of jokes and also have a chuckle with the patient

- Do something loving towards yourself each day - the simplest gesture is rewarding such as using a beautifully fragrant oil in your bath, watching your favourite TV programme, munching something delicious whilst dipping into a delightful book, exercising to jolly music, contemplating a beautiful flower

- Regular visits to the hairdresser and/or beautician

- Regular massage and facials

- Keeping the home environment comfortable and pleasant

- Finding travel organisations who cater for disabled people so that appropriate holidays or short breaks may be taken

- Attend activities at Caregivers support groups

Chapter 35

Helpful Contacts

Disclaimer: The Authors and Publisher cannot be held responsible for the outcome of any advice given by the following independent contacts.

- *Stress Relief Techniques - Exercise*
    – Mobility/Lifestyle
- *Healthy Soaps*
- *Bookshops - Nutritional Supplements*
- *Caregivers' Associations*
- *Parkinson's Support Associations*
- *Holiday Assistance – Flying Without Fear*

STRESS RELIEF TECHNIQUES

CD Recording: "Parkinson's Disease – Relaxation" ISBN - 10: 0-9551661-0-1
ISBN - 13: 978-0-9551661-0-5 by David Uri, DHP FAPHP MNCH NGH(USA) FRSH
Fellow of The Royal Society of Medicine, London UK
Email: **da**videuri@yahoo.co.uk

Orders: www.amazon.co.uk and bookshops

Autogenic Training Courses in London, UK
The Royal Homeopathic Hospital
Greenwell Street, London W1W 5BP
Website: **www.autogenic-therapy.org.uk**

Galin Tudhope BA Psych MSc LCD Dip AT (Autogenic Training/Psychotherapy)
Email: **Ga**ylin@5tconsulting.net

EXERCISE

Adrienne Golembo (Building Better Backs and Bodies), London, UK
T: **07973 122615**
Email: **adri**enne@b4backs.co.uk
Website: **www.b4backs.co.uk**

SOAPS (SKIN AND HOUSEHOLD), (no harmful additives)
Droyt Soap Company
Website: www.droyt.com

Bio-D (Household Cleaning Products)
Website: http://www.biodegradable.biz.

MOBILITY/LIFESTYLE PRODUCTS (UK)
Hearing and Mobility
Website: https://www.hearingandmobility.co.uk/

BOOKS (USA) (all genres and health)
Amazon.com
Website: www.amazon.com

Barnes and Noble (USA)
Website: www.bn.com

Borders (USA)
Website: www.borders.com

BOOKS(UK) (nutrition, general health and self-help)
Order at all bookshops

Amazon.co.uk (all genres)
Website: www.amazon.co.uk

NUTRITIONAL SUPPLEMENTS (UK)
The Natural Dispensary
Website: www. Naturaldispensary.co.uk

CAREGIVERS ASSOCIATIONS (USA) include
Parkinson's Resource Organisation:
Email: info@parkinsonsresource.org
Website: www.parkinsonsresource.org

Michael J Fox Foundation
Website: https://www.michaeljfox.org/

National Parkinson's Disease Foundation Inc.
Website: http://www.parkinson.org/

CAREGIVERS ASSOCIATIONS (UK) include

Carers Trust
Website: https://carers.org/

The National Care Association
Website: http://nationalcareassociation.org.uk/

European Parkinson's Disease Association:
Website: http://www.epda.eu.com/

UK Parkinson's Disease Society
Website: https://www.parkinsons.org.uk/

PARKINSON'S DISEASE ASSOCIATIONS WORLD-WIDE

AUSTRALIA
Parkinson's Australia:
Website: http://www.parkinsons.org.au/

WESTERN AUSTRALIA
Parkinson's Western Australia
Website: https://www.parkinsonswa.org.au/

AUSTRIA
Parkinson Selbsthilfeverein Oberosterreich

BELGIUM
Belgische Parkinson Vereniging

BRAZIL
Website: http://www.parkinson.org.br/firefox/index.html

CANADA
The Parkinson's Foundation of Canada
Website: www.parkinson.ca

CHILE
Liga Chilena Contra el Mal de Parkinson
Website: http://parkinson.cl/

CZECH REPUBLIC
Společnost PARKINSON, z. s/ Czech Parkinson's Disease Society
Website: http://www.parkinson-brno.cz/

DENMARK
Dansk Parkinson Forening/ Parkinsonforeningen
Website: http://www.parkinson.dk/

EUROPE
European Parkinson's Disease Association
Website: www.epda.eu.com

FAEROES
Parkinsonfelagið
Website: http://www.parkinson.fo/

FINLAND
Suomen Parkinson-liitto ry
The Finnish Parkinson Association
Website: https://www.parkinson.fi/

FRANCE
FFGP - Fédération Française des Groupements de Parkinsoniens
Website: http://assoffgp.wixsite.com/ffgp

Association France Parkinson
Website: http://www.franceparkinson.fr/

GERMANY
Deutsche Parkinson Vereinigung Bundesverband e.V.
Website: https://www.parkinson-vereinigung.de/start

ICELAND
PSÍ - Parkinsonsamtökin á Íslandi
Website: http://parkinson.is/

INDIA
Parkinson's Disease and Movement Disorder Society
Website: http://www.parkinsonssocietyindia.com/

IRELAND
Parkinson's Association of Ireland (including PALS Support Group for Younger People)
Website: http://www.parkinsons.ie/

ISRAEL
Israel Parkinson Association
Website: http://www.parkinson.org.il/

ITALY
Parkinson Italia (ONLUS)
Confederazione Associazioni Italiane Parkinson E Parkinsonism
Website: http://www.parkinson-italia.it/

JAPAN
Movement Disorder Society of Japan
Website: http://www.movementdisorders.org/MDS/AOS-Partners/Movement-Disorder-Society-of-Japan.htm

LUXEMBOURG
Parkinson Luxembourg (PL) a.s.b.l
Website: http://www.parkinsonlux.lu/

MEXICO
Asociacion Mexicana De Parkinson A.C.
Website: https://ampacmexico.com/

NETHERLANDS
Parkinson Vereniging (PV)
Website: https://www.parkinson-vereniging.nl/

NEW ZEALAND
The Parkinsonism Society of New Zealand
Website: http://www.parkinsons.org.nz/

NORWAY
Norges Parkinsonforbund
Schweigaardsgt. 34, bygg F, oppg. 2, Oslo 0191, Norway
T: **+ (47) 22-175-861**
Fax: **+ (47) 22-175-862**

PERU
Asociacion Peruana Para La Enfermedad De Parkinson

SLOVENIA
Društvo TREPETLIKA/ Parkinson's Disease Society of Slovenia
Website: http://www.trepetlika.si/

SOUTH AFRICA
South African Parkinson Association
Website: www.parkinsons.co.za/

SPAIN
Federación Española de Párkinson/ Spanish Federation of Parkinson Disease
Website: http://www.fedesparkinson.org/

SWEDEN
ParkinsonFörbundet/ The Swedish Parkinson's Disease Association
Website: http://www.parkinsonforbundet.se/

SWITZERLAND
Parkinson Schweiz
Website: http://www.parkinson.ch/

TAIWAN
Taiwan Movement Disorder Society
Website: http://www.movementdisorders.org/MDS/AOS-Partners/Taiwan-Movement-Disorder-Society.htm

THAILAND
Movement Disorder Society of Thailand
Website: http://www.movementdisorders.org/MDS/AOS-Partners/Movement-Disorder-Society-of-Thailand.htm

UNITED KINGDOM
The Cure Parkinson's Trust, UK
Website: https://www.cureparkinsons.org.uk/

European Parkinson's Disease Association
Website: http://www.epda.eu.com/

Parkinson's UK
Website: https://www.parkinsons.org.uk/
Y.A.P.P.&.R.S. (Young Alert Parkinson's Partners & Relatives)
Email: enquiries@parkinsons.org.uk

"Movers & Shakers" is committed to driving momentum towards a cure through high-impact profile-raising initiatives and by generating funds for The Cure Parkinson's Trust, UK.
Website: http://www.pdoutreach.org/

Parkinson's Disease Nurse Specialist Association (PDNSA)
Website: http://www.pdnsa.org/

Parkinson's Disease Nurse Specialist Association (PDNSA) Website:
pdnsa.org.com

UNITED STATES
Parkinson's Resource Organisation:
Website: http://www.parkinsonsresource.org/

Parkinson's Disease Foundation (PDF)
Website: http://www.pdf.org/

National Parkinson's Disease Foundation Inc. (NPF)
Website: http://www.parkinson.org/

The American Parkinson Disease Association (APDA)
Website: https://www.apdaparkinson.org/

Michael J Fox Michael J Fox Foundation
Website: https://www.michaeljfox.org/

Movement Disorder Society (MDS):
Website: https://www.movementdisorders.org/MDS.htm

Continued over page ➥

ASSISTED TRAVEL (world-wide)

The Assistance Travel Service Ltd (ATS Travel)
T + 44 (0) 1708 863198
Website: http://www.assistedholidays.com

FEAR OF FLYING (specialised courses and self-help book)

Virgin Atlantic Flying Without Fear (UK courses) UK bookings:
T: 01423 714900

International bookings:
T: + 44 1423 714900
Email: info@flyingwithoutfear.info
Website: www.flyingwithoutfear.info
(for books and courses)

Index

X
Stevia, 84

Z
Zandopa HP200, 34 (monitoring), 66,99
Zelapar, 32, 52
Zinc
- body function, 7, 8
- carbonic anhydrase, 10, 11
- deficiency evidence, 24
- foods containing, 99
- hydrochloric acid and protein
    digestion, 10, 11
- insulin, 13
- intravenous nutrition, 122
- iron, 21
- male sexual health, 142
- superoxide dismutase, 22, 62
- supplement, 22
- test, 15